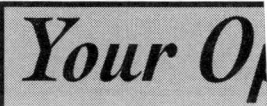 

Cosmetic Surgery

Jane Smith BSc (Hons)
Medical Editor and Writer, Bristol

&

John Kenealy MBChB, FRACS (Plas)

Consultant Plastic Reconstructive and Aesthetic Surgeon,
Frenchay Hospital, Bristol;
Honorary Consultant Plastic Reconstructive and
Aesthetic Surgeon, Southmead Hospital, Bristol;
and Senior Clinical Lecturer in Surgery,
University of Bristol

ILLUSTRATIONS BY ALEXANDER JAMES

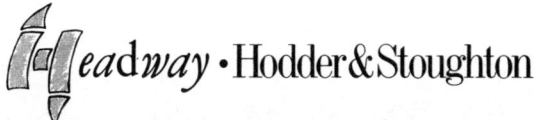

Other titles published in this series

Breast Lumps
Hernias
Hysterectomy & alternative operations
Varicose Veins
Male and Female Sterilisation
Cataracts
Skin Cancers
Prostate Problems
Hip Replacement
Knee Replacement

A catalogue record of this publication is available from the British Library.

ISBN 0 340 664460

First published 1997
Impression number   10 9 8 7 6 5 4 3 2 1
Year   2002   2001   2000   1999   1998   1997

Copyright © 1997 Jane Smith

All rights reserved. No part of this publication may be reproduced or transmitted in any form or by any means, electronic or mechanical, including photocopy, recording, or any information storage and retrieval system, without permission in writing from the publisher or under licence from the Copyright Licensing Agency Limited. Further details of such licences (for reprographic reproduction) may be obtained from the Copyright Licensing Agency Limited, 90 Tottenham Court Road, London W1P 9HE.

Typeset by Wearset, Boldon, Tyne and Wear.

Printed in Great Britain for Hodder & Stoughton Educational, a division of Hodder Headline Plc, 338 Euston Road, London NW1 3BH, by Cox & Wyman Ltd, Reading, Berks.

Contents

General preface to the series		vi
Preface		ix
Acknowledgements		x
PART I	**GENERAL CONSIDERATIONS**	1
Chapter 1	**Asking questions and making choices**	3
	Who has cosmetic surgery?	4
	Why have cosmetic surgery?	4
	The role of your family doctor	6
	How to choose your surgeon	7
	Questions to ask the surgeon	9
	Cosmetic clinics	10
	Getting the operation you want	11
	When surgery is refused	12
Chapter 2	**Discussions and decisions**	14
	Reasons for having cosmetic surgery	14
	Reasons why surgery may be inadvisable	16
	Pre-operative appointments	17
	Pre-operative tests	19
	Making the decision	20
Chapter 3	**Going in to hospital for an operation**	21
	What to take in to hospital	22
	Hospital staff	24
	Admission to the ward	28
	Pre-operative procedures	29

	The anaesthetic room	33
	The operating theatre	34
PART II	**THE OPERATIONS**	**35**
Chapter 4	**The face, neck and brow**	**37**
	Retinoeic acid creams	37
	Chemical peel	38
	Dermabrasion	39
	Laser dermabrasion	40
	Face and neck lift	41
	Brow lift	47
Chapter 5	**The eyes**	**50**
	Blepharoplasty	50
Chapter 6	**The nose**	**57**
	Rhinoplasty	57
Chapter 7	**The lips**	**62**
	Collagen injections	62
	Goretex	63
	Surgical techniques	64
Chapter 8	**The ears**	**65**
	Pinnaplasty	65
Chapter 9	**The breasts**	**69**
	Breast implants	69
	Breast augmentation	70
	Breast reduction	76
	Breast lift	81
Chapter 10	**Fat removal**	**82**
	Liposuction	82
	Abdominoplasty	86
	The treatment of cellulite	91

CONTENTS

PART III	**GENERAL RISKS AND COMPLICATIONS OF SURGERY**	**93**
Chapter 11	**Possible post-operative complications**	**95**
	Pyrexia	96
	Bruising	96
	Pain	96
	Bleeding	97
	Wound infection	98
	Necrotising fasciitis	98
	Wound dehiscence	99
	Skin necrosis	99
	Fluid collection	99
	Scarring	99
	Nerve damage	100
	Chest infection	101
	Deep vein thrombosis	101
	Pulmonary embolism	102
APPENDICES		**103**
Appendix I	**Anaesthesia and pain relief**	**105**
	Local anaesthesia	105
	General anaesthesia	106
	Side-effects of general anaesthesia	108
	Risks of general anaesthesia	108
	Patient-controlled analgesia	109
Appendix II	**Paying for your operation**	**111**
	Private health insurance	111
	Paying for your operation yourself	112
Appendix III	**Case histories**	**114**
Appendix IV	**Medical terms**	**120**
Appendix V	**Useful addresses**	**136**
Appendix VI	**How to complain**	**140**
Index		**145**

General preface to the series

Two people having the same operation can have quite different experiences, but one feeling that is common to many is that things might have been easier if they had had a better idea of what to expect. Some people are reluctant to ask questions, and many forget what they are told, sometimes because they are anxious, and sometimes because they do not really understand the explanations they are given.

In most medical centres in Britain today, the emphasis is more on patient involvement than at any time in the past. It is now generally accepted that it is important for people to understand what their treatment entails, both in terms of reducing their stress and thus aiding their recovery, and of making their care more straightforward for the medical staff involved.

The books in this series have been written with the aim of giving people comprehensive information about each of the medical conditions covered, about the treatment they are likely to be offered, and about what may happen during their post-operative recovery period. Armed with this knowledge, you should have the confidence to question, and to take part in the decisions made.

Going in to hospital for the first time can be a daunting experience, and therefore the books describe the procedures involved, and identify and explain the roles of the hospital staff with whom you are likely to come into contact.

Anaesthesia is explained in general terms, and the options

GENERAL PREFACE TO THE SERIES

available for a particular operation are described in each book.

There may be complications following any operation – usually minor but none the less worrying for the person involved – and the common ones are described and explained. Now that less time is spent in hospital following most non-emergency operations, knowing what to expect in the days following surgery, and what to do if a complication does arise, is more important than ever before.

Where relevant, the books include a section of exercises and advice to help you to get back to normal and to deal with the everyday activities which can be difficult or painful in the first few days after an operation.

Doctors and nurses, like members of any profession, use a jargon, and they often forget that many of the terms that are familiar to them are not part of everyday language for most of us. Care has been taken to make the books easily understandable by everyone, and each book has a list of simple explanations of the medical terms you may come across.

Most doctors and nurses are more than willing to explain and to discuss problems with patients, but they often assume that if you do not ask questions, you either do not want to know or you know already. Questions and answers are given in most books to help you to draw up your own list to take with you when you see your family doctor or consultant.

Each book also has a section of case histories of people who have experienced the particular operation themselves. These are included to give you an idea of the problems which can arise, problems which may sometimes seem relatively trivial to others but which can be distressing to those directly concerned.

Although the majority of people are satisfied with the medical care they receive, things can go wrong. If you do feel you need to make a complaint about something that happened, or did not happen, during your treatment, each book has a section which deals with how to go about this.

It was the intention in writing these books to help to take some of the worry out of having an operation. It is not knowing what to expect, and the feeling of being involved in some process over which we have no control, and which we do not fully understand, that makes us anxious. The books in the series *Your Operation* should help to remove some of that anxiety.

You may not know *all* there is to know about a particular condition when you have read the book related to it, but you will know more than enough to prepare yourself for your operation. You may decide you do not want to go ahead with surgery. Although this is not the authors' intention, they will be happy that you have been given enough information to feel confident to make your own decision, and to take an active part in your own care. After all, it is *your* operation.

Jane Smith
B*ristol*, 1997

Preface

This book has been written to provide clear, comprehensive information for anyone contemplating cosmetic surgery. It covers the most common cosmetic operations and deals primarily with *surgery* rather than with the non-surgical techniques that can be used to treat some problems when surgery is inappropriate. It stresses the importance of finding out all you can about what your operation entails and about the experience, training and qualifications of the surgeon who is to perform it, as well as the need to have realistic expectations about what can be achieved. When you have read this book, you should be able to approach discussions with your surgeon with confidence, knowing what questions you want to ask and how to interpret the answers you are given to them.

Part I of the book contains three chapters that are of relevance to anyone contemplating any type of cosmetic surgery. They explain the factors that should be considered before deciding to go ahead with an operation, and give details of the various pre-operative procedures common to most type of cosmetic surgery. Chapters 4 to 10 in Part II describe what is likely to happen before, during and after the various operations, and the specific complications that can occur. Part III contains only one chapter (Chapter 11), which should be read by everyone, whatever type of cosmetic operation they are considering. It explains the potential complications associated with any type of surgery. Although very serious complications are relatively rare, it is important to be aware of what could go wrong so that you can seek medical advice and receive any necessary treatment at an early stage.

The appendices include details of the different types of anaesthesia that may be used; how to go about paying for your operation; some brief case histories; explanations of common medical terms you may come across; some useful addresses; and the best way to approach any complaint that may arise in relation to the operation you have had.

Jane Smith
John Kenealy
B*ristol*, 1997

Acknowledgements

We are particularly grateful to Judith Hine-Haycock, RGN, Plastic Surgery Practice Sister and Plastic Surgery Theatre Nurse Specialist, Bristol, for her helpful comments. Thanks are also due to the members of staff at the BUPA Hospital, Bristol, who spared the time to discuss various aspects of caring for patients undergoing cosmetic surgery; and to the women who shared their experiences with us for the section of case histories.

PART I

General considerations

The chapters in this part of the book are relevant whatever type of operation you are considering. They will help you to compile your own list of questions to ask your surgeon, to make informed decisions about the treatment you require, and to have an understanding of the various routine pre-operative hospital procedures and hospital staff you are likely to encounter.

CHAPTER 1

Asking questions and making choices

Some cosmetic operations have been performed since the early 1900s, but the wide range available today has been made possible by the advances in surgical techniques that have occurred since then, particularly in recent years.

Any operation which is truly 'cosmetic' clearly cannot be considered to be medically essential, and it is therefore vital that anyone contemplating this type of surgery understands all that is involved and has realistic expectations of what can be achieved.

Cosmetic surgery is increasingly becoming an option for 'ordinary' men and women; most popular magazines carry advertisements for cosmetic clinics and private hospitals. (Individual surgeons are not permitted to advertise.) But it is important to understand that all cosmetic operations are *surgical* procedures – not 'beauty parlour' treatments – and although many people are happy with the results of their surgery, things can go wrong. As with any type of surgical procedure and the use of an anaesthetic, there are potential risks that have to be borne in mind before making a decision to go ahead with cosmetic surgery.

The purely *aesthetic* operations with which this book is mainly concerned are not usually available in the UK under the National Health Service (NHS). However, some operations undertaken to correct congenital abnormalities (i.e. those present since birth) or deformities resulting from accidents or other forms of injury can be done under the NHS system in some areas of the country, depending in part on local policy.

WHO HAS COSMETIC SURGERY?

In 1995, approximately 65 000 cosmetic operations were performed in the UK and 3 million in the USA, the majority for women, although the number of men undergoing cosmetic surgery is gradually increasing.

Like it or not, Western society places significant emphasis on physical appearance. One only needs to look at the huge income derived from the cosmetics industry and from fashion to realise that many people are prepared to spend money (sometimes quite substantial sums) to look as good as they can. It is little wonder, then, that cosmetic surgery is becoming a more acceptable and more popular way of making long-lasting, if not permanent, changes to people's appearance.

Even if you are not a film star or television personality, whose livelihood depends to some extent at least on what you look like, you may have been unhappy for many years with a particular physical characteristic that seems to you to be 'abnormal' or simply at odds with how you would like to see yourself. It is therefore not just the rich and famous who undergo cosmetic surgery, but people from a wide spectrum of life with very varied incomes.

The operations described in this book are rarely suitable for children, especially before they have finished growing in their mid to late teens. However, an exception to this is pinnaplasty – a reconstructive rather than purely cosmetic operation to correct the congenital abnormality of prominent ears (see p.65).

WHY HAVE COSMETIC SURGERY?

Western society does not generally revere the attributes of age and many people fear not only old age itself, but also the signs that it is approaching. Some therefore seek cosmetic surgery to reverse the physical signs of ageing. Others wish to alter a particular physical characteristic to make them look more 'normal' or attractive.

Reversing the signs of ageing

This type of cosmetic surgery is done for a variety of reasons: because people wish to look younger, and thus feel more attractive, or because they feel that their position in their workplace will become less secure as they age. For example, older men and women who feel their jobs are threatened by young, ambitious colleagues may feel that by looking more youthful they can increase their chances of competing.

Altering an 'abnormal' physical feature

In medical terms, the spectrum of what constitutes an 'abnormal' feature has more to do with function than appearance, but to the average person the category is far wider.

Although most cosmetic operations are done privately, it is sometimes possible to have surgery under the NHS in the UK to correct a congenital abnormality or one which a surgeon considers to be causing psychological distress. However, in areas where NHS treatment is available, waiting lists tend to be long. Even so, before exploring private surgery, it may be worth asking your doctor's advice about the local criteria for, and availability of, NHS treatment.

Sometimes, operations are done to relieve physical symptoms such as the chronic backache that can result from very large breasts and which can be treated by breast reduction (see p.76).

Typecasting

The assumptions and prejudices associated with certain physical 'types' can make life difficult for someone who does not fit the mould. For example, not all men with misshapen noses get involved in fights, and not all women with large breasts wish to be seen as sex symbols! Therefore, some people seek cosmetic surgery in an attempt to alter a physical feature they feel colours other people's attitudes towards them.

THE ROLE OF YOUR FAMILY DOCTOR

In theory, plastic surgeons based at NHS and private hospitals prefer patients to be referred to them by their family doctors. In practice, many people approach surgeons directly, and this is certainly the case at most cosmetic clinics. In the latter situation, before going ahead with surgery, the surgeon may contact your doctor to request details of your medical history or of any other relevant factors, such as allergies, any adverse reaction you may have had to an anaesthetic used at a previous operation, any medical condition from which you suffer, including diabetes, heart or respiratory disease, and any medication you are taking. Occasionally, however, family doctors who are unsympathetic to patients seeking cosmetic surgery decline to provide this information, in which case the surgeon will have to decide whether or not to go ahead without it. If, for some reason, you do not wish your family doctor to be contacted, you should tell your surgeon, who may offer you counselling about your reasons for this request. But it is always best to approach your family doctor at the outset to discuss the cosmetic surgery you want to have and to ask for a referral to a reputable and experienced surgeon.

If your doctor is unwilling to arrange a referral, your local NHS or private hospital will be able to provide the names of accredited aesthetic plastic surgeons with private practices who undertake the type of operation you are considering – although staff at the hospital will not wish to recommend any particular surgeon. You can then telephone the secretary of the surgeon of your choice and ask for an appointment; this may also be a good time to ask about the surgeon's experience and qualifications (see below).

It is essential that you feel comfortable with the surgeon you choose and with other members of the hospital or clinic staff, and there is no reason why you should not discuss your operation with several surgeons before making the decision to go ahead.

HOW TO CHOOSE YOUR SURGEON

Surgery that goes wrong, or that does not achieve the desired effect, can lead, at best, to disappointment and, at worst, to complications that may or may not be correctable by further surgery. It is therefore important to reduce the risks by choosing a competent, appropriately trained and experienced surgeon.

In most countries, including the UK and the USA, there is little real regulation of the practice of cosmetic surgery. In theory, any qualified doctor in the UK can decide to practise as a cosmetic surgeon, even one who has had no previous experience of this specialty other than some undergraduate surgical training. You therefore need to find out about your surgeon's qualifications, training and experience *before* agreeing to undergo any type of cosmetic operation.

Most cosmetic surgery is done at private hospitals, cosmetic clinics and, in the UK, in private wards within NHS hospitals. In the UK, the majority of surgeons with private practices also work for the NHS, and are therefore likely to have many years of surgical experience. However, *general* surgical experience alone does not equate with competence in a particular specialty, and it is therefore helpful to know how much *appropriate training* a surgeon has. The General Medical Council (GMC) operates a *specialist register* of surgeons in the UK who have accredited training in particular specialties, including plastic surgery (see Appendix V).

Although a surgeon's qualifications are important, they are

only significant if you understand what they mean. In Britain, although it would be difficult to obtain the qualification Fellow of the Royal College of Surgeons (FRCS) without some surgical experience, the examinations involved are theoretical rather than practical and are usually taken within four years of first qualifying as a doctor. Once a doctor has become 'FRCS', he or she can then go on to train in a particular surgical specialty, such as cardiac, orthopaedic or plastic surgery etc. To become a qualified plastic surgeon, for example, and obtain the qualification FRCS (Plas), involves undergoing *specialist training* in plastic surgery and passing further examinations. Surgeons in Britain may also be members of the British Association of Plastic Surgeons (BAPS) and/or of the British Association of Aesthetic Plastic Surgeons (BAAPS), both of which denote training in *plastic* surgery and peer acceptance of suitable qualifications. A suitably qualified plastic surgeon is likely to be a Board Certified Plastic Surgeon in the USA.

When you telephone to make an appointment with a particular surgeon, you can also take the opportunity to ask about his or her training and qualifications. For example, is the surgeon an accredited plastic surgeon? Does he or she have any area of special surgical interest? As you can choose your surgeon, it seems sensible to choose one with particular experience of the specific operation you wish to have.

You should also rely to some extent on your own instincts when choosing a surgeon: do you feel able to talk freely to him or her and think that you will have a good, workable relationship? Do not forget that you are *choosing* to have surgery for aesthetic reasons – it is not necessary as a life-saving procedure – and you must be confident that you will receive skilled, competent and sympathetic care. There is no reason why you should not make appointments with two or three surgeons before making your choice.

QUESTIONS TO ASK THE SURGEON

Wherever you have your operation, do not feel embarrassed to ask the surgeon as many questions as you think necessary; your questions may also help to reassure the surgeon that you have considered your operation carefully and are taking a sensible interest in all matters relating to it.

You should be able to put all your questions directly to the surgeon, rather than to nurses or non-medical staff. If you are encouraged to make an instant decision about surgery, you probably have good reason to suspect that your operation may be being viewed primarily in financial terms.

The following points will probably be dealt with during your consultation with the surgeon, but you may want to ask about anything that remains unclear.

* *What is involved in the operation and what are the results it is hoped can be achieved?* A surgeon who glosses over full discussion of *all* aspects of the operation is probably not the best person to perform it.
* *What are the major complications in relation to your particular operation and are they correctable – by medical or surgical means?* Surgeons who perform any type of surgery, however competent and experienced they may be, are almost bound to encounter some difficulties at some time, but they should be happy to discuss the potential problems with their patients.
* *Has the surgeon received training, in a certified training programme, to do the operation being considered?* Bear in mind, though, that apart from surgeons with appropriate training in plastic surgery, there are some very competent specialists in other fields who perform some cosmetic operations – for example ear, nose and throat (ENT) surgeons may perform operations to correct 'bat ears' etc.

  The answer to this question will provide you with more

information than simply asking how many times the surgeon has performed a particular operation – which does not tell you whether he or she does it well!

You will have to rely to some degree on your own feeling of confidence in the surgeon when interpreting the answers to these questions.

If you are having your operation at a private hospital or cosmetic clinic, you may also want to ask:

* *What emergency facilities are available?* NHS hospitals have specialist nurses and doctors trained in emergency procedures and able to deal with any medical emergencies that might arise. Even the best-planned operations, performed by the most competent surgeons and anaesthetists, can go wrong, for example if a patient has an undetected heart condition or an allergy to the anaesthetic used. It is therefore essential to find out whether trained staff and a full range of emergency equipment will be on hand to deal with these sorts of problems.

After your first consultation, a reputable surgeon may suggest you take some time to think about your operation and will want to be sure that you are well-informed and happy with your decision.

COSMETIC CLINICS

Cosmetic surgery has become 'big business' and there are now many cosmetic clinics and many very experienced, highly qualified surgeons practising in them. But there are also some surgeons and some clinics that are less reputable and, in the UK, the level of competence is probably more variable in cosmetic clinics than it is in NHS and private hospitals. Therefore, if your operation is being done at a cosmetic clinic, it is particularly important to ask the right questions and satisfy yourself that you will receive appropriate care.

As already mentioned above, you would be wise to be wary of any clinic where less attention is paid to addressing your concerns and providing comprehensive information than it is to encouraging you to sign up for surgery as quickly as possible.

GETTING THE OPERATION YOU WANT

Apart from your general state of fitness and health, there are various factors the surgeon will need to take into account before deciding to go ahead with your operation.

There are both anatomical and functional constraints on what it is possible to do – you will need to be able to breathe through your reshaped nose! The relative proportion of certain of your physical features will also need to be considered by the surgeon, who may suggest an alternative to the operation you are seeking. For example, it may be suggested that, rather than having the size of your nose reduced, your chin is built up in order to keep the two features in balance. Or you may be advised to have a brow lift as well as eyelid surgery if drooping of your brow has caused extra tissue to be pushed into your upper eyelid. If you are having a face lift, and perhaps liposuction or lipectomy of the neck, and have a flat chin, it may be suggested that you also have a chin implant to avoid emphasising a 'turkey gobbler' neck.

It is important that you and your surgeon agree about the aim of the operation. For example, if you wish to have the size of your nose reduced, do you both have the same idea of what your reshaped nose should look like? If you are contemplating breast reduction, does the surgeon know what size (i.e. cup size) you want your new breasts to be?

It is therefore vital to discuss fully with the surgeon the effect you hope will be achieved and to make sure you understand what the surgeon thinks can be done. It is no good discovering after your operation that you each had a quite different understanding of what was required. However, it should also be borne in mind that it is almost impossible for any surgeon to know exactly what the results of an operation will be as they may be influenced by factors such as the quality of your bone and tissue – which will not become apparent until surgery is underway (or even afterwards) – and the effects of post-operative scarring.

An additional consideration is that everyone's physical features are unique: a nose which suits one person will look quite different on someone else. Therefore, although you may wish to show the surgeon a photograph of someone with a nose you admire, you must be prepared to accept that you would probably look quite different, even were it to prove possible to alter the shape of your nose in exactly the same way. You are thus far less likely to suffer disappointment after your operation if you have a clear idea of precisely what it is you *dislike* about the physical feature you wish to have altered, rather than precisely what you want it to look like.

A good surgeon will discuss all these aspects with you.

WHEN SURGERY IS REFUSED

Before agreeing to operate, your surgeon will want to make sure that your reasons for requesting cosmetic surgery are appropriate (see p.15), and that you do not have exaggerated expectations of the outcome or of the personal or psychological problems it will cure. Therefore it is very important to take note of any doubts expressed by the surgeon and, if necessary, to give serious thought to any suggestion that an operation would be inappropriate. If a surgeon turns down your request for surgery, it is tempting simply to look elsewhere for someone who *will* do the operation. But it really is in your own best interests to accept what a reputable surgeon tells you and to think again about whether you really need or want surgery.

In some circumstances, surgeons suggest referring people to a psychologist to discuss their reasons for wanting cosmetic surgery (see p.17).

CHAPTER 2

Discussions and decisions

Even if you have already decided to go ahead with surgery, it is a good idea to think about exactly what you hope can be achieved by it, both physically and in terms of the effect it may have on your life. It is important to be honest with yourself, and to make sure your aspirations are realistic.

Following most types of cosmetic surgery, there will be a period of anything between a few days and several weeks during which the operated area will be inflamed and bruised, possibly quite severely. Therefore, you should decide in advance how you will cope with this, and be prepared to take some time off work and/or use make-up or some other means of camouflage.

Do not expect to leave hospital after your operation looking and feeling wonderful; it may be several weeks or more before the full effects become apparent. If you have a general anaesthetic (see p.106), you may feel a little unwell and possibly a bit depressed for at least a day or two.

REASONS FOR HAVING COSMETIC SURGERY

If you visit your family doctor in the first instance, he or she may be very sympathetic and supportive, but this is not always the case. If you have already made up your mind to have cosmetic surgery, a negative reaction from your doctor may not deter you, but do make sure that you listen to any specific points raised during the discussions you have.

No cosmetic operation can be a panacea for all life's problems and a good doctor or surgeon will want to be sure that you would not be better served by non-surgical treatment, counselling or some other form of support. There are therefore several factors that need to be taken into account, both by doctors and the individuals concerned. It is surprising how easy it is to be swept away by enthusiasm at the prospect of cosmetic surgery without considering some basic points.

For cosmetic surgery to be appropriate, you should have:

* a desire for a change in your appearance, rather than trying to satisfy someone else's idea of how you should look;
* a real desire to have the operation, as well as realistic apprehension about it;
* a defect that is obvious to both you and the surgeon;
* realistic expectations about what can be achieved by the operation, both physically and with regard to changes in your personal life;
* no medical condition or other contraindication that could complicate surgery or your recovery from it;
* a clear understanding of what the operation involves, the possible complications, and the length of time you will have to spend in hospital and recovering at home afterwards;
* no psychological contraindication to surgery;
* sufficient funds to pay for the operation.

You should also be able to take enough time off work to recover from your operation, and should have help and support at home while you are unable to do household chores, drive, lift heavy objects and, if relevant, look after your children. You may need to ask for help from friends, even if you do not wish them to know the reason why.

Only if you meet all these requirements should you really be considering cosmetic surgery.

REASONS WHY SURGERY MAY BE INADVISABLE

If the surgeon you talk to expresses doubts about undertaking the operation you request, it could be for one or more of the following reasons.

* You want to reduce your apparent age by an unrealistic number of years, for example 20 or 30.
* You wish to look the same as you did many years previously, perhaps in an old photograph.
* You are convinced that surgery will resolve some problem in your personal life or lead to promotion at work.
* You are seeking surgery to please someone other than yourself.
* You are obese and think that surgery such as liposuction or an abdominoplasty will be an easy way of 'losing weight'.
* You wish to have a complete 'overhaul' and undergo several cosmetic operations to change your appearance drastically: it could well be that some aspect of your life other than your physical appearance needs to be changed.
* You do not know exactly what it is you wish to alter, and have rather vague ideas about the surgery you want.
* Your desire to have cosmetic surgery has been precipitated by a trauma in your life, such as divorce or the death of someone close to you.
* You have already had a cosmetic operation but the outcome was not what you had hoped for and you think further surgery will result in the desired (possibly unrealistic) effect.

As has already been mentioned, except in exceptional circumstances, cosmetic surgery is rarely appropriate for children. It is also usually advisable for parents to wait until their children can make their own decisions about whether or not to have a particular physical feature altered.

The role of the psychologist

Although many people find that cosmetic surgery has a positive effect on their lives and psychological well-being, it is not always the right answer. If the surgeon thinks there may be more effective ways of dealing with an underlying cause of dissatisfaction or unhappiness, it may be suggested that you talk to a psychologist before making a decision. This would not indicate that the surgeon has doubts about your sanity! It may simply be that she or he feels that cosmetic surgery may not be the right answer for you. If this option is suggested, it is worth approaching it with an open mind, as spending a large sum of money on an operation that fails to deal with the true cause of your problem could simply add to it.

PRE-OPERATIVE APPOINTMENTS

At your pre-operative appointment, the surgeon will examine the feature you wish to have altered, and will ask you various questions, as outlined above. The operation itself, its probable outcome and any potential complications should also be explained to you.

Whatever type of cosmetic operation you are having, the surgeon will question you about your medical history, about any factors that could increase the risk of anaesthesia or surgery, and possibly about any illnesses and/or causes of death of your near relatives. It is important to mention *any* health problems you have, or have had in the past, as they could have a relevance of which you are unaware. Although an existing medical condition will not necessarily preclude you from having surgery, the surgeon needs to know about it to be able to take any necessary precautions before, during and after your operation.

If you have had any problems in the past such as an allergy to a particular anaesthetic, it will be helpful if you know the name of the drug concerned and/or the hospital where the operation was carried out so that the appropriate records can be checked and another type of anaesthetic given to you. You should also tell the surgeon if any other member of your family has reacted against a particular anaesthetic drug, as you may have the same problem.

It is a good idea to write down anything that occurs to you, however trivial it may seem, and take your note with you when you visit the surgeon. It is also helpful to make a note of any specific questions you wish to ask, as you may not remember them at the time.

You may have a second appointment with the surgeon before your operation to discuss precisely what needs to be done. Do make sure that you are quite clear about what the surgeon plans to do, and about the expected outcome of the operation.

If you are taking a contraceptive pill, you will probably be advised to stop doing so for six weeks before your operation, during which time you should use an alternative method of contraception. Although the modern contraceptive pills contain quite low doses of hormone – particularly compared to earlier ones – it is thought that they can increase the post-operative risk of **thrombosis** and blood clots (**thrombi**, see p.101).

Recent reports have suggested that hormone replacement therapy (HRT) may be linked to a small increased risk of **thrombo-embolism** – the breaking off of a fragment of a blood clot which then blocks the passage of blood through a blood vessel, with potentially serious consequences. However, although there is no evidence to indicate that the risk is any greater in women undergoing surgery, some surgeons ask their patients to stop taking HRT for a period pre-operatively.

You should tell the surgeon about all other drugs you have been taking, including any of which your family doctor may be unaware, such as vitamin supplements, cough medicines, aspirins etc. that are available from a pharmacy without the need for prescription.

PRE-OPERATIVE TESTS

Although pre-operative tests are rarely performed routinely before cosmetic surgery, some may be done if there is clinical suspicion of a problem, such as a heart or chest condition.

* *X-rays*. A chest X-ray may be done to detect any lung abnormality that could complicate the use of a general anaesthetic or that will need to be treated before or after surgery.
* *Electrocardiogram*. If there is any reason to think that you may have a cardiovascular problem, an electrocardiogram (ECG) may be done so that the surgeon and anaesthetist can take any necessary precautions during and after surgery.

  Electrodes are taped to the wrists, ankles and skin over the chest to record the pattern and size of the electrical waves produced by the muscles of the heart as it beats. An abnormal pattern indicates some dysfunction of the heart, such as a poor blood supply, abnormal rhythm or weak heart muscle. It is important to lie as still as possible during the few minutes it takes to do an ECG so that electrical impulses generated by the movement of other muscles do not mask those from the heart.

  Throughout any operation done using a general anaesthetic, electrodes from a similar ECG monitor are attached to the patient's chest to make sure the heart rhythm remains normal.
* *Blood tests*. Oxygen, which is essential for the health and repair of the tissues of the body and for wound healing, is transported in the blood attached to haemoglobin. If your haemoglobin level is low pre-operatively (i.e. you are anaemic), it will fall even further when blood is lost during surgery. Therefore, a sample of your blood may be taken to measure its haemoglobin level and, if this is found to be low, you may be prescribed a course of iron tablets to bring it up to normal.

Blood transfusions are rarely necessary for most types of cosmetic operation, but if there is thought to be a chance you may need a transfusion for any reason, your blood may be cross-matched to make sure you receive blood of the correct group.

If appropriate, your blood will also be tested for sickle cell anaemia or thalassaemia.

* *Urinalysis.* A sample of your urine may be analysed if there is suspicion of diabetes or renal disease.

MAKING THE DECISION

Once a surgeon has agreed to do the operation you have requested, it is up to you to decide whether or not to go ahead with surgery. If at any stage you feel that you are being put under pressure, or you do not have complete confidence in your surgeon, make an appointment to talk to another surgeon before making your decision. If you develop *any* doubts, ask for your operation to be cancelled or postponed to give yourself time to reconsider, regardless of how late in the proceedings you have changed your mind.

If you feel comfortable with your surgeon, are aware of all that is involved in the operation, including the potential complications, and if you are clear about your reasons for wanting surgery, you can go ahead knowing that you have done everything possible to ensure you make an informed decision.

CHAPTER 3

Going in to hospital for an operation

Some cosmetic operations can be done as day-case surgery (see below); others involve a night or two in hospital post-operatively.

This chapter gives general details of the hospital procedures and of the medical staff you are likely to come across. Although most people having cosmetic surgery are treated privately, a few in the UK receive treatment under the NHS. Where relevant, any differences between the two systems are mentioned.

You should receive from the hospital or clinic a letter telling you the date of your operation and any other details you need to know, and may also be sent a pre-admission form to fill in and take with you when you are admitted, and a leaflet explaining the admission procedures. The time of your admission depends on the normal practice at your particular hospital.

> **Day-case surgery** Day-case surgery is being used increasingly for straightforward operations, and is suitable for several types of cosmetic surgery. The average cost of an operation involving an overnight stay in hospital is considerably greater than the cost of the same operation done as a day case.
>
> You may be admitted to hospital only an hour or two before your operation, and may be able to leave almost immediately after surgery if you have a local anaesthetic, or within a few hours if you have a general anaesthetic.
>
> If you require any pre-operative tests (see p.19), they may be done by your family doctor a week or two before surgery, or at a pre-operative appointment at the hospital.

WHAT TO TAKE IN TO HOSPITAL

For day-case surgery, you may want to take your own slippers, dressing gown and washing things into hospital (see below), but otherwise you will only need something to read or to keep yourself occupied during periods of waiting. If you are staying in hospital overnight or longer, the following list may be helpful.

1 *Nightclothes*. You may be given a hospital gown to wear during your operation. You will be able to dress again after day-case surgery, but will need your own nightclothes if you are staying in hospital overnight.
2 *Slippers*. You will need slippers to wear after your operation when you return to your hospital ward or private room, and some people prefer to wear them before and after day-case surgery too.
3 *Dressing gown*. You will need a dressing gown to wear on the ward, and some day-case patients also like to wear one on the way to the operating theatre.
4 *Towel and washing things*. You will need your own washing things for an overnight stay in hospital, and may wish to take them with you to have a wash before you go home after day-case surgery.
5 *Money*. If you are being treated at a private hospital or clinic, the cost of newspapers and telephone calls etc. will be added to your bill. If you are being treated under the NHS, a *small* amount of money may be useful to pay for these.

Large sums of money, wallets and handbags should never be taken into hospital; in an NHS hospital they may have to be kept in an unlocked cabinet beside your bed. If for any reason you do have to take any jewellery, valuables or large sums of money into hospital, they should be given to the ward sister for safe keeping when you are admitted. Each item will be listed on a receipt, which will be given to you and which you will need to produce when you collect your possessions on leaving hospital. However, it is always better to make arrangements for any valuables you do not wish to leave at home to be looked after by a relative or friend while you are in hospital.

6 *Books, magazines, puzzles, knitting etc.* There will inevitably be periods of waiting between visits from medical staff before your operation, and you may want something to occupy you during this time.

7 *Drugs you are already taking.* You may be asked to take with you into hospital any drugs you normally need so that their dosages can be checked and so that you can continue to be given any which are necessary. All your drugs will be kept for you during your stay, as you must only take those that are given to you by medical staff. Any drugs you do take into hospital should be returned to you before you leave.

If you are being treated under the NHS, your family doctor will have been asked to fill in a form stating all the drugs you are taking and their doses.

8 *Admission letter.* An admission letter will have been sent to you from the hospital or clinic (and probably from the surgeon too), and you should take this with you when you are admitted for your operation.

Wedding rings Wedding rings, or any other rings that are very precious to you or that cannot be removed, will be covered with adhesive tape before your operation. This is to prevent the metal causing burns during the process of **diathermy** that is used to stop the little blood vessels bleeding. One type of diathermy often used, **bipolar diathermy**, involves passing an electric current through the two prongs of a pair of forceps to produce localised heat between them, to seal the ends of blood vessels.

HOSPITAL STAFF

Hospitals are busy places and can seem rather confusing and frightening. It may help to have an idea of the different medical staff you are likely to meet, and the jobs they do. The following details are based on current practice in the UK; the roles and titles of medical staff in other countries will differ slightly.

Nurses

The uniforms worn to distinguish nurses of different ranks vary from hospital to hospital, but all nurses wear badges that state clearly their name and sometimes their grade. There are, of course, both male and female nurses, although women are still in the majority.

Apart from the ward staff mentioned below, there are also various other nursing staff who work in particular areas of hospitals such as the operating theatre and recovery room. *Operating theatre nurses* are qualified nurses who have gone on to specialise in surgery and who assist, and work closely with, surgeons during operations. *Recovery room nurses* are qualified, specially trained nurses who care for patients coming round from anaesthetics after operations.

1. The most senior nurse on a ward is the *ward sister* or *ward manager*. Each ward will have one ward sister, who will be very experienced and able to answer any questions you may have. The ward sister has 24-hour/day responsibility for all the staff and patients on at least one ward, for the day-to-day running of the ward, standards of care etc., and is ultimately responsible for the ward even when not on duty. The ward sister will be a registered nurse (RN) or a registered general nurse (RGN), who has usually been qualified for at least five years. Ward sisters may wear a uniform of a single colour, often dark blue.

The male equivalent of the ward sister is a *charge nurse*, whose rank will be clearly displayed on his name badge.

2 When the ward sister is not on duty, there will be a *senior staff nurse* or a *team leader* of another grade in charge. The senior staff nurse is deputy to, and works closely with, the ward sister and, like her, will be very experienced.

3 Each ward may have several *staff nurses*, who may be newly qualified or may have several years' experience, and who will take charge of the ward when both the ward sister and senior staff nurse are unavailable. There are different grades of staff nurse, distinguished by different coloured belts, epaulettes, uniforms or, more rarely nowadays, hats.

The majority of staff nurses on an NHS ward are likely to be junior staff nurses, who are very often in their first or second post since qualifying, and who are less involved in ward management and therefore able to work closely with the patients. Most nurses working in private hospitals are likely to be more senior.

4 *Enrolled nurses* are gradually being replaced and can now undergo a training programme to become staff nurses, with the qualification of RGN. However, there are still many enrolled nurses working on NHS hospital wards who are very experienced and sometimes team leaders (see above). They have undergone two years of training and, like the junior staff nurses, are mainly involved in patient care rather than ward management.

5 *Health care assistants* (HCAs) are unqualified nurses who have undergone six months' training on day release while working on a ward and who have then been assessed for a National Vocational Qualification (NVQ) by senior nurses. They are supervised at all times by a qualified nurse and are able to carry out all basic nursing duties except for the dispensing of drugs. Health care assistants are being brought in to work in NHS hospitals to take the place of student nurses, who now spend more time in college and less on hospital wards.

6 The ward may also have several *nursing auxiliaries* to deal with any non-medical jobs and to help with the basic care of patients such as making beds, serving tea, and putting away linen etc. Although nursing auxiliaries are not trained nurses, some are very experienced and have acquired greater responsibility.

7 Student nurses – *diploma nursing students* or P*roject* 2000 *students* – are unpaid and allocated to the wards of NHS hospitals at various stages during their college-based training. They are mainly involved in observing and carrying out limited clinical tasks. In their last term before they qualify, they are rostered on to nursing shifts to be part of a ward team. Student nurses do not work in private hospitals or clinics.

Doctors

Most private hospitals employ resident medical officers who are fully qualified, registered doctors, available 24 hours a day to deal with any emergencies that may arise. However, this is not necessarily true of all cosmetic clinics (see p.10).

If your operation is being done privately, it will be performed by the surgeon you have already met, but this may not be the case if you are being treated under the NHS.

1 *Consultant surgeons* have at least 10 years' surgical experience. Those employed by the NHS hold the ultimate responsibility for all the patients on their operating lists, and for the work of all the doctors in their team. However, if you are being treated under the NHS, you may not actually see the consultant surgeon who is responsible for your care, although you should be visited on the ward before your operation by whichever surgeon is to perform it.

2 A *senior registrar* is an experienced surgeon who has completed several years of training and will soon be appointed to a consultant post. An NHS operation may be performed by a senior registrar. (This grade is soon to be phased out.)

3 Some NHS operations are performed by *registrars*. Registrars have trained as surgeons for at least two or three years and are able to carry out some surgery alone, assisting the consultant, or being assisted by the consultant, on more difficult operations.

4 Some NHS hospitals employ *clinical assistants* or *staff grade doctors*, often very experienced surgeons who, for personal or family reasons, are not able to work full time, or who are family doctors with surgical experience.

5 If you are being treated under the NHS, you may be examined before your operation by a *senior house officer* (SHO) or by a house surgeon (see below). Senior house officers have been qualified doctors for between one and five years, and are gaining further experience in hospital before becoming surgeons or specialising in another branch of medicine. They may perform some minor operations in NHS hospitals.

In private hospitals, senior house officers are the doctors on call to deal with emergencies.

6 *House surgeons* (or *house officers*) do not work in private hospitals, but may be directly concerned with the care of NHS patients both before and after their operations, taking notes of their medical history and arranging for any necessary preoperative investigations to be done, such as blood tests, chest X-rays or electrocardiograms. (As has already been mentioned, if you are receiving private care, all these details will be dealt with by your consultant.)

House officers are qualified doctors who have completed at least five years of undergraduate training and are working for a further year in hospital before becoming fully registered doctors. Although they do not perform surgery on their own, they may assist the surgeon in the operating theatre.

In addition to the surgical staff listed above, an *anaesthetist* may also be involved in your care while you are in hospital. Anaesthetists are doctors who have trained in the administration of drugs that cause loss of sensation and/or consciousness (anaesthetics) and those that block feelings of pain (analgesics).

ADMISSION TO THE WARD

When you arrive at a private hospital or clinic, you should report to the main reception desk with your admission letter. The staff there will check your details, and a ward receptionist will come to collect you and show you to your room, which is likely to be a single or double room with a private bathroom, telephone and television. If you are paying for your operation yourself, you will probably be asked to pay your bill in advance at this stage, if you have not already done so.

If you are being treated under the NHS, you will be told which ward to go, where a ward clerk or nurse will deal with the clerical side of your admission, filling in the necessary forms with you. You will then be shown to your bed and told of any ward details such as meal times, where to find the toilets, day room etc. A **named nurse** will be allocated to you and will admit you to the ward, look after you during your stay, and co-ordinate your discharge when the time comes. (You will be allocated another nurse for other working shifts.) You may be asked to help your nurse draw up a care plan and should tell her of any ailments, preferences or dislikes you have, for example if you prefer to sleep with several pillows or if there are certain foods you do not like. The nurse may discuss your discharge arrangements with you at this stage and, if you are having a general anaesthetic, will want to be sure that you will have someone to care for you at home until its effects have worn off. The ward sister will, of course, be informed of all aspects of your care, and will be able to discuss it with you or your relatives.

In private hospitals and clinics, where each nurse is usually responsible for the care of fewer patients than in NHS hospitals, the use of 'named nurses' is not necessary.

PRE-OPERATIVE PROCEDURES

Your blood pressure, temperature and pulse will be measured and a sample of your urine may be taken for analysis to make sure you do not have diabetes or any disorder of the kidneys that could complicate the operation. You may also be weighed if the anaesthetist needs to know your weight in order to be able to calculate the dose of anaesthetic you require.

After certain types of operation there is a risk of thrombosis (see p.101), and precautions may be taken to reduce this risk, particularly if your mobility is likely to be restricted for any length of time.

Anti-embolism stockings

Anti-embolism stockings (often called TEDS – **t**hrombo-**e**mbolic **d**eterrent **s**tockings) are thought to help prevent blood clots forming in the veins deep within the legs by improving the return of venous blood to the heart (see p.101). They are used routinely in some hospitals, but are not normally necessary for people having local anaesthesia or very brief operations.

If you do need to wear anti-embolism stockings, a nurse will measure your calf, thigh and the length of your legs once you are settled on the ward. If you have a history of varicose veins or thrombosis that increases your risk of developing a blood clot, you will probably have to wear the stockings throughout your hospital stay. Otherwise, you may not need to put them on until you are preparing to go to the operating theatre and can remove them once you are mobile again after surgery.

Heparin injections

Anyone with a previous history of thrombosis, or who is otherwise at increased risk of developing blood clots, may be given injections of low-dose heparin during their stay in hospital. Heparin is an **anticoagulant** drug which occurs naturally in the body and helps to thin the blood and prevent it clotting.

Visit by a doctor

Private patients are visited by their consultant surgeons before their operations. A house surgeon or senior house surgeon, and possibly the surgeon who is to perform the operation, will probably visit NHS patients pre-operatively.

> **Consent forms** You will be asked to sign a consent form declaring that your operation has been explained to you and that you understand what it entails and have agreed to it taking place. You are also giving your permission for the doctors to take whatever action they feel to be appropriate should some emergency occur during surgery, and for any necessary anaesthetic to be given to you. Do read this form carefully *before you sign it*, and ask the doctor to explain anything you do not understand.

Visit by the anaesthetist

Local anaesthetics are usually injected by the surgeon rather than by an anaesthetist. But if you are having a general anaesthetic, the anaesthetist will probably come to see you after you are admitted to hospital to discuss your general health and to ask about anything that may be relevant to the choice of anaesthetic, any anaesthetics you have had before, and any drugs you are taking. It is important that you answer these questions as fully as possible so that you are given the anaesthetic that is safest for you. Do talk to the anaesthetist about any problems or worries you have concerning your anaesthesia.

Pre-medication

Anaesthetics have improved considerably in recent years, and the routine use of pre-meds. is now rare. However, if you or your anaesthetist feel that you are very anxious and need something to relax you, you may be given some form of sedative, by mouth or injection, about an hour before surgery (probably while you are still on the ward), which will soon make you feel sleepy.

Other medication

The anaesthetist will explain about other tablets and drugs that may be required before your operation for any reason, for example antibiotics or blood-thinning drugs. You may also be given any drugs that you normally take, such as diuretics ('water tablets') or drugs to reduce high blood pressure.

> **General anaesthesia and driving** The effects of general anaesthetic gases, and other agents used by the anaesthetist, can stay in your body for several days, and although you may feel you are fully recovered, your reaction times will be slow and you may continue to feel sick and light-headed for at least a day or two. It is therefore important that you *do not attempt to drive yourself home* when you are discharged from hospital.
>
> You should also bear in mind that you are unlikely to be covered by your normal car insurance for some time after having a general anaesthetic or intravenous sedation. Someone at your insurance company will be able to tell you how long this restriction lasts.

False teeth

You should tell the anaesthetist if you have any false teeth or dental bridges as these will have to be removed before you go into the operating theatre to avoid a broken or loose tooth being inhaled into the lungs during surgery. You should also point out any teeth that are crowned. At some hospitals, patients are able to keep their false teeth in place until they reach the operating theatre, rather than having to take them out on the ward.

'Nil by mouth'
This term means that neither food nor drink must be swallowed. If you are having a general anaesthetic, you will be told not to eat or drink anything for four to six hours beforehand to prevent you vomiting and to avoid the risk of choking on your vomit while you are anaesthetised. You will be able to have a few sips of water with any tablets you need to take, and some anaesthetists now allow their patients to drink clear fluids up to three hours pre-operatively.

Waiting

Long delays and the postponement of operations are uncommon in private hospitals and cosmetic clinics, where there are rarely emergency admissions to deal with and where the nurse to patient ratio is usually higher than in NHS hospitals.

The pre-operative wait is likely to be a little longer for NHS patients. Apart from having to be seen by all the medical staff mentioned above, who are responsible for many other patients as well, time may also have been allowed for the assessment of any medical problems you may have, and for the results of blood tests etc. to be received.

Cancellation of operations

In NHS hospitals, operations sometimes have to be cancelled at the last moment if an emergency has arisen or an earlier operation has taken longer than expected. If this occurs, you may be sent home, but every effort should be made to admit you again at the earliest opportunity.

Although cancellation of your operation would be very distressing, and possibly awkward if you have had to arrange child care and/or time off work, do try not to get upset. Urgent operations cannot be postponed.

Cancellation of operations happens only rarely at private hospitals.

Leaving the ward for your operation

Before being taken from the ward to the anaesthetic room or operating theatre, you will be given a hospital operating gown to wear. A plastic-covered bracelet bearing your name and an identifying hospital number will be attached to one or both of your wrists. You will then be taken from the ward on a hospital trolley or on the bed from your room, although if you are having a local anaesthetic, you may be able to walk to the operating theatre or be taken in a wheelchair.

You will be asked several questions to confirm your identity and to make sure that you are ready for the operation. These questions may be repeated several times by different people: many people have many types of operation each day in a hospital and checks are essential to make sure no mistakes are made.

THE ANAESTHETIC ROOM

For some types of cosmetic operation, only the operating site itself is anaesthetised, by the injection of local anaesthetic, the effects of which last for a limited period of time. Local anaesthetic can often be administered by the surgeon in the operating theatre.

Other operations require a general anaesthetic, which anaesthetises the whole body and some of the effects of which may last for several hours. The anaesthetic drugs will be introduced into your body through a small tube called a **cannula**, which the anaesthetist will insert into a vein in the back of your hand, and which will be kept in place throughout the operation. Cannulas are often inserted routinely whatever type of anaesthetic is being used. (General anaesthesia is explained in more detail in Appendix I.)

An important member of the anaesthetic team is the *operating department assistant* (ODA), a highly skilled technician who assists the anaesthetist both before and during operations. An ODA will probably carry out several of the pre-operative procedures in the anaesthetic room (see p.106).

THE OPERATING THEATRE

You will be taken from the anaesthetic room into the operating theatre, where you will be lifted from the hospital trolley on to the operating table and positioned appropriately for your particular operation. Before the operation starts, the operating site will be cleaned with an antiseptic solution.

PART II

The operations

Chapters 4 to 10 describe what will happen before, during and after the various operations dealt with, and explain the specific complications that can occur in each case.

Some operations can now be performed endoscopically, and the following brief explanation describes what is involved in this technique.

> **Endoscopic surgery** With the recent advances in technology and in the manufacture of surgical instruments, have come advances in surgical techniques, and mention is made in individual chapters of operations for which endoscopic surgery may be appropriate.
>
> An endoscope is a flexible, fibre-optic telescope that contains a bright light source and a channel through which surgical instruments are inserted and manipulated. Once the endoscope has been introduced into the body through an incision, the surgeon can view the operation on a video or television monitor in the operating theatre as he or she performs it.
>
> Although the incisions made during surgery performed endoscopically are smaller than those required for conventional surgery, it is the distribution of scars rather than the total amount of scarring that differs between the two techniques.

CHAPTER 4

The face, neck and brow

Skin becomes less elastic with age, and muscles and connective tissue tend to lose their tone. The results in the face and neck are deepening of the folds around the mouth and eyes, drooping of the corners of the mouth, sagging of the jaw line, and loosening of the folds of skin on the neck. (The loss of a significant amount of weight can also produce similar effects.) The age at which these changes start to become visible is partly genetically determined, but is also dependent on factors such as diet, general health and fitness. Excessive sun exposure, smoking and some illnesses also affect the quality of the skin.

Although this chapter deals primarily with surgical procedures, there are also several non-surgical facial treatments to help improve the general quality of the skin, some of which can be carried out at the same time as a face lift (see p.41). Following all of these non-surgical procedures, the skin is very sun sensitive and must be protected with a high-factor sunscreen. The most common of these treatments are described below.

RETINOEIC ACID CREAMS

There are various creams (for example Retin A and Retinova) containing a substance called tretinoin, derived from vitamin A, that can reduce some of the signs of sun damage such as brown spots and fine wrinkles, although they can cause swelling, itching, burning and peeling of the skin to begin with. The creams should not be used by anyone with eczema or spider veins, as they can exacerbate these conditions; due to the increased sun sensitivity they cause, they are also unsuitable for anyone with a history of skin cancer.

The creams work by encouraging the production of new cells in the lower layer of the epidermis of the skin, and by increasing the rate at which dead cells are shed from the skin's surface. They may also improve the elasticity of the skin by increasing its production of collagen. It may be three or four months before any visible effects of treatment are apparent, and individual satisfaction with the results varies.

Daily treatment should continue for at least six months, a small amount of cream being applied each night after washing the face. Thereafter, any improvement can be maintained by using the cream two or three times a week. If treatment is stopped, the effects already obtained may last for a year or two.

Normal make-up and skin creams can be used during treatment, although astringent cleansers should be avoided. The regular use of a moisturiser will help counteract the dryness caused by retinoeic creams.

Retinoeic creams are available on private prescription from family doctors, plastic surgeons and dermatologists.

CHEMICAL PEEL

A chemical peel has an effect similar to, although less dramatic than, dermabrasion (see below). It involves the use of corrosive chemicals (usually trichloroacetic acid, or phenol for a deeper peel) rather than the surgical instruments used to remove the outer layer of skin in dermabrasion. Great care is needed to ensure that the chemical does not penetrate too deeply below the surface layer of the skin and cause scarring – although this sometimes cannot be avoided. Chemical peels are usually most successful for people with fair skin.

Some specialists advise the use of retinoeic cream (see above) on the face each day for about four weeks before a chemical peel, and some advise the use of a bleaching solution. Clear instructions will be given; do make sure you understand them and follow them precisely.

Chemical peels are usually done at an out-patient clinic. The type of anaesthetic used will depend to some extent on the depth of the peel: a local anaesthetic or anaesthetic cream may be sufficient, but a deep peel using phenol requires a general anaesthetic or deep sedation.

The skin is wiped with alcohol to remove its natural oil before the chemical substance is painted on and allowed to set. The resulting 'mask' may be left until it drops off spontaneously, or may be peeled away. The skin is then bathed with an iced saline solution to reduce pain and is covered with petroleum jelly.

The treated skin can remain red for three months or more, but the application of a prescribed steroid cream may help reduce this redness and control itching.

DERMABRASION

Dermabrasion is a surgical procedure for smoothing the skin. It is usually done as day-case surgery (see p.21) using either a local or general anaesthetic. One technique involves the use of a small rotating instrument to remove the outer skin layer from the face, and with it any blemishes, fine lines or shallow scars. However, now that the risks of HIV and AIDS have become a matter of concern, this type of dermabrasion is no longer common and will probably eventually be superseded by laser skin resurfacing (see below).

After dermabrasion, the skin is painful and may bleed for several days; regular pain-killing tablets may be required for about two weeks. A scab will start to form a couple of days or so after treatment, and will probably fall off after eight to ten days. The skin beneath the scab will be a livid red colour, which will gradually fade over the next three months or so.

LASER DERMABRASION

Also known as **laser skin resurfacing**, this process involves the use of special carbon dioxide lasers to remove a very thin layer from the surface of the skin to improve its texture and reduce fine facial wrinkling and some deeper wrinkles, particularly crows' feet and wrinkles around the mouth. It is probably less effective for the removal of deeper furrows, for example on the forehead. More recently, ERBIUM:YAG lasers have been introduced, which provide even more superficial resurfacing and give good results when used to reduce very fine wrinkles.

The depth of penetration of the laser can be precisely controlled, allowing for a more consistent removal of tissue than is achieved with a chemical peel or mechanical dermabrasion – and therefore a reduction in some of the risks associated with the latter methods.

Laser dermabrasion may be combined with blepharoplasty (see p.50) to improve the appearance of lightly wrinkled and/or bulging lower eyelids and avoid external scars. It can also sometimes enhance the effect of a mini face lift (see p.42), but is not a substitute for a full face lift as it does not *lift* the facial tissues.

Laser dermabrasion is not a painless procedure and requires the use of anaesthetic, either a local or topical anaesthetic for the treatment of small areas, or deep sedation or a general anaesthetic for larger areas.

Following laser treatment, the surface of the skin is raw. It may be covered with dressings or left open to heal spontaneously, over approximately seven to ten days, depending on the depth of the tissue removed. The new skin is likely to be pink or red for a few weeks, possibly less so following treatment with ERBIUM:YAG lasers than is likely with carbon dioxide lasers. On rare occasions, redness can remain for several months, during which time it can be concealed by make-up.

Laser dermabrasion also tightens the skin – an effect that does not seem to occur following a chemical peel or mechanical dermabrasion. This tightening takes place several months after healing, and can continue for up to a year, so that the resurfaced skin often looks better at 12 months than it did at two months after laser treatment.

The risks of laser dermabrasion are similar to those of other methods, and include an increase or decrease in pigmentation or patchiness, and scarring.

FACE AND NECK LIFT

Any operation to tighten the skin of the face, which may also involve tightening and sometimes repositioning of the soft tissues beneath the skin, is known as **rhytidectomy** – literally, the removal of wrinkles. This type of surgery can remove some of the visible signs of ageing and/or neglect and is most successful when done between the ages of 40 and 60, when the skin and muscles are still in reasonably good condition. A first face lift performed after the age of 60 is likely to be less effective as the skin and muscles will already have lost their tone and elasticity. The ageing process continues after surgery, and therefore the effects of a face lift will not last forever, although the operation can usually be repeated when required. The results of rhytidectomy will vary from person to person.

Before your operation

During a pre-operative appointment, the surgeon will examine (and possibly take photographs of) your face and neck. You will be questioned about your medical history and general health, and any necessary pre-operative tests will be arranged for you (see p.19).

If you plan to lose weight, you should do so *before* you have a face lift so that the resulting excess skin can also be removed. You may wish to visit your hairdresser before your operation as you will not be able to have your hair permed or coloured for a few weeks afterwards, until the small scars have healed and will not be irritated by the chemicals used in these processes. You may be advised to wash your hair with a special shampoo the night before surgery.

The operation

There are several slightly different types of face-lift operations which can be done – including the mini lift, composite lift, mask lift, endoscopic lift and SMAS lift – and your surgeon will choose the one that is most appropriate for you. The SMAS face lift is probably the most common of these procedures in the UK, and involves not only the skin but also a layer of soft tissue and muscle beneath it known as the superficial musculo-aponeurotic system, or SMAS layer.

The following is a general description of the basic techniques involved in all face-lift operations. Most are performed under general anaesthetic, although occasionally local anaesthesia and sedation may be used.

Once the anaesthetic has taken effect, an incision is made in the skin, starting at the hairline just behind the temple and running down immediately in front of the ear. In most cases, the incision passes behind the small extension of cartilage near the earhole (known as the **tragus**), although occasionally, especially for men, it runs in front of it. It is then continued around the earlobe, up behind the ear, across the bare skin overlying the mastoid process (the hard bit of bone that can be felt behind the ear), and usually ends up in the hairline again. Sometimes the final part of the incision is made along the base of the hairline.

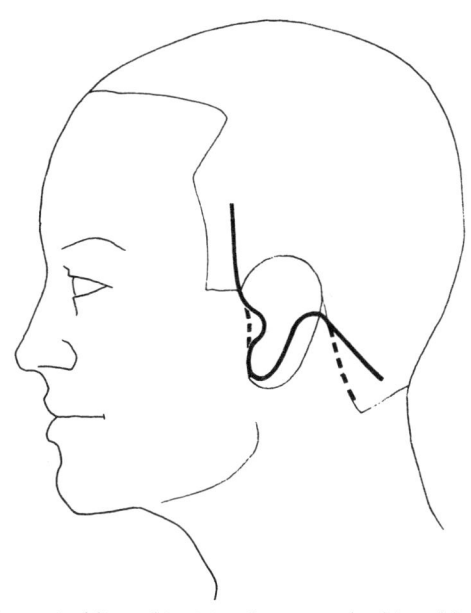

Face lift. The typical line of incision for a standard face lift. The dashed lines show alternative routes, the one passing in front of the tragus of the ear often being used for men.

The skin, together with a very thin layer of fat, is then separated from the underlying tissues, sometimes extending as far forward as the **nasolabial fold**, the area between the nose and the upper lip. The dissection of skin is also continued down to the neck and, if significant neck lifting is needed, may be carried further forward in the neck. The dissected skin and fat are then tightened (by being pulled backwards and slightly upwards) and the excess is cut away.

The SMAS lift

The operation described above results in improvement in skin laxity but does not affect the drooping (known as **ptosis**) of the soft tissues that frequently occurs with age. Therefore, when the underlying soft tissues in the SMAS layer need to be tightened to correct ptosis, the SMAS face lift is more appropriate. It involves either taking tucks and pleats in the SMAS layer (a process known as **plication**), or dissecting the SMAS as a separate layer and tightening it in much the same way as the overlying skin is tightened but with more upward pull. The excess skin is then removed and a drainage tube may be placed underneath the repositioned skin before it is stitched back in place.

Surgery to one side of the face is usually completed before the same procedure is started on the other side. A light dressing may then be applied to the face.

The mask lift

The surgical technique of a mask lift is similar to that described for the SMAS lift, but involves lifting *all* the facial structures – soft tissues and muscles – to a depth just above the bone.

The endoscopic lift

A mask lift can sometimes be partly performed endoscopically through several small incisions in the scalp and lower eyelids. The technique is relatively new and not all surgeons have experience of this operation, which is therefore not available at all hospitals and clinics. Its efficacy is still being evaluated and debated.

The composite lift

This is a far more extensive operation, involving lifting of the face, brow (see p.47) and upper eyelids (see p.52).

After your operation

When you come round from the anaesthetic, your face may be bandaged and there is likely to be at least one small drainage tube inserted under the skin to remove the blood and fluid which collect there. The drain(s) will probably be removed within about 24 to 48 hours, or when drainage reduces, and the dressings after one to five days. Your hair might be washed the day after your operation, and your wounds redressed.

Although rhytidectomy is not a particularly painful operation, it can be uncomfortable. Bruising may be severe and will last for at least a couple of weeks; swelling may remain for longer. The facial skin may itch and feel tight, and headaches may persist for several days. There is likely to be numbness in the cheeks, neck and area around the ears, which can last for three months or more.

For the first few days after a face lift, you should keep your head upright as much as possible, and may find it helpful to sleep on several pillows. Make-up can usually be used about four days after a face lift, but should not be put on the skin near stitches or small wounds. Until the stitches (and clips, if used) have been removed, probably within about a week after surgery, you should try to avoid moving your head suddenly to the side. All sports and other strenuous activities should be avoided for at least a couple of months. You may need at least three weeks off work, partly to allow time for the worst of the bruising and swelling to subside. You may continue to feel very tired for some time after your operation.

Before you leave hospital, you will be told how to wash your hair – using a *mild* shampoo. Although the wounds will probably close within about 48 hours after surgery, you should not allow them to become soaked with water, or hang your head down forwards, until they have healed completely, and some doctors therefore advise waiting at least ten days before hair washing. It will be three weeks or more before you can have your hair permed or coloured.

However well prepared you think you are before your face lift, you may be quite depressed by your appearance in the first few days after surgery. The regular use of analgesic tablets will help control any pain, and a determinedly positive attitude will assist you during the days when you look much worse than you did before your operation! Depending on the type of face lift you have had, it may be two to six months before the signs of surgery have disappeared and you can see any real improvement.

Possible complications

Most of the complications that can occur after face-lift surgery can do so after any type of operation (see Chapter 11). Occasionally, the nerves that control the movement of the mouth and eyebrows suffer some degree of damage, and may take six weeks or longer to recover. Rarely, some nerves fail to repair themselves, leading to permanent loss of movement in the affected area, for example at the corner of the mouth. The more extensive the dissection, the greater the risk of temporary or permanent injury being caused to branches of the facial nerve, and of complications such as skin loss or haematoma (see p.97).

Any hair which has been lost around the incisions made in the scalp usually grows back within about three weeks, although occasionally it never does so. There will always be a tiny bald spot around each scar, which should be quite easy to conceal.

Other possible complications include the development of spider veins on the face, and permanent hyperpigmentation of patches of bruised skin. Asymmetry of the face may occur as a result of differences in the healing of the two sides but may respond to revision.

Sometimes scars fail to fade over the months, but as they are mostly hidden in the natural creases around the ears, they should be fairly inconspicuous. Rarely (most commonly in smokers), skin necrosis may occur (see p.99), resulting in scarring in prominent areas, for example on the cheek following a face lift and on the neck after a neck lift. Once the scar has had time to settle, it may be possible for its appearance to be improved surgically.

Some people are disappointed with the results of their face lift, often because they do not look as young as they had hoped. This is usually the result of unrealistic expectations or of limitations due to the quality of their tissues. Laser resurfacing (see p.40) or a chemical peel (see p.38) may lead to further improvement.

BROW LIFT

There are two groups of muscles in the forehead that control the raising and lowering of the eyebrows. As these muscles weaken with age, gravity tends to cause the brows to droop. This effect can be counteracted by surgery to cut the muscles which lower the eyebrows and to elevate the skin. However, any existing furrows or horizontal lines on the forehead cannot be completely eradicated by a brow lift, although they may be further reduced by a subsequent chemical peel (see p.38) or laser treatment (see p.40).

Brow lifts can be done using a local anaesthetic and sedative or general anaesthesia. They are not normally performed as day-case surgery. If other facial surgery is done at the same time, an overnight stay in hospital will probably be necessary.

Before your operation

The usual details will be noted by the surgeon at your pre-operative appointment (see p.17) and your face and brow will be examined carefully. Any necessary tests will be arranged for you (see p.19).

The operation

Brow-lift surgery can either be performed using conventional techniques or endoscopically (see p.35).

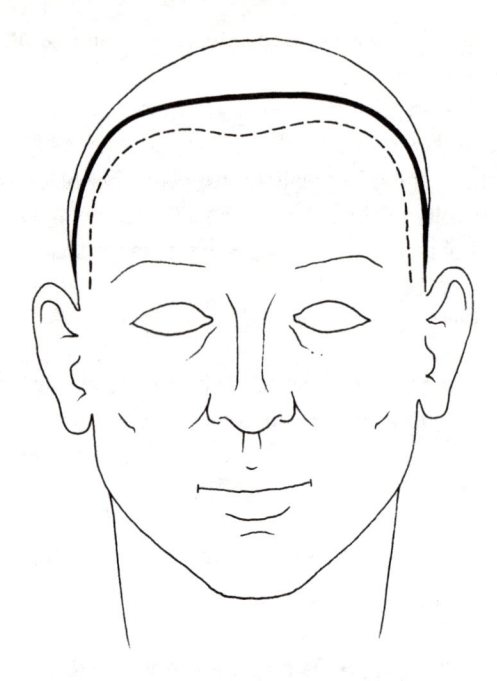

Brow lift. The typical line of the incision made across the scalp. The dashed line shows an alternative route along the margin of the hairline that may be used for someone with a high forehead.

For a conventional brow lift, the surgeon makes an incision within the hairline, extending from one temple to the other. If the hairline is high, this incision may be made at its margin to avoid further lengthening of the forehead. The skin and muscle of the forehead are then lifted off the underlying skull, as far down as the supraorbital rim above the eyes, and pulled tight. Between 1.5 and 2.5 cm (about 0.5 and 1 inch) of excess skin is cut away, and the remaining skin is repositioned and secured with stitches. In the course of this procedure, any overactive muscles causing forehead creases and frown lines may be resected or divided.

For an endoscopic operation, the surgeon makes multiple smaller incisions vertically in the hairline and performs the dissection under endoscopic control. As less skin is resected when this technique is used, fixation of the elevated brow is more difficult. Therefore, the skin is often secured with special surgical glue or (rarely) screws. The long-term efficacy of endoscopic brow lifts is still being debated.

After your operation

Any stitches used to close the incisions will be removed after about four to seven days. Bruising around the eyes and along the cheeks may take a few weeks to fade completely, and you may experience a tingling sensation in your forehead, and possibly numbness for about a week. Once the numbness resolves, you should be able to move your eyebrows again. Any hair lost from around the incisions should grow back within about three months, although occasionally it never does so.

Possible complications

Apart from the general complications described in Chapter 11, the specific complications that can occur after brow-lift surgery are similar to those of a face lift (see p.46). The main additional risks are overcorrection, so that the eyebrows are permanently raised, and asymmetry of the two eyebrows.

CHAPTER 5

The eyes

Records of eyelid surgery date back to the early tenth century in Arabia, when operations were performed to improve impaired vision by excising excess skinfolds in the upper eyelid. Surgical techniques have continued to improve since that time, particularly during the last century, and an operation known as **blepharoplasty** is now commonly undertaken to reduce the effects of ageing by removing excess skin and fat from the upper and lower eyelids, or to correct congenital or familial abnormalities.

BLEPHAROPLASTY

The effects of blepharoplasty are likely to last for many years, although the operation can be repeated if necessary. Blepharoplasty is sometimes performed as day-case surgery, using a local anaesthetic and sedative, but if it is done at the same time as a face lift, a general anaesthetic is normally used. However, some surgeons prefer all their patients to stay in hospital overnight after eyelid surgery to monitor for haematoma (see p.97) or the rare complication of loss of vision postoperatively (see p.55).

Before your operation

Although the eyes themselves are not involved in eyelid surgery, it is important to tell the surgeon about any existing eye problems or any previous eye surgery you have had. Some surgeons advise anyone contemplating blepharoplasty to undergo a routine eyesight test.

At a pre-operative appointment, the surgeon will examine your eyelids to make sure that blepharoplasty is the most appropriate way of dealing with your problem; sometimes excessive skin in the upper eyelids is better corrected by a brow lift (see p.47). Your visual acuity and tissue elasticity will be tested, and the surgeon will make sure your tear production is adequate to reduce the risk of dry eyes after surgery.

You will be questioned about your medical history and general health: surgery may not be appropriate for those with various medical conditions such as hyperthyroidism and hypothyroidism. Any pre-operative tests thought to be necessary (see p.19) will be arranged for you.

The operations

Apart from the two main operations described here, additional procedures may be carried out as required to accentuate the fold in the upper eyelid, thin the muscle to reduce activity in the lower eyelid, and tighten and lift the outer corner of the eye.

Upper eyelid blepharoplasty

Incisions are made through the skin and muscle, and an ellipse of skin is excised from a site in the upper eyelid such that the resulting scar is hidden in the natural eyelid crease. The **orbicularis oculi muscle**, which lies underneath the skin, is split between its fibres, and in some cases muscle is resected to allow the formation of a skin crease. There are two compartments of fat under the muscle, bulging of which is often responsible for puffiness around the eyes. Excess fat is removed from these compartments and care is taken to seal any small blood vessels before the skin is stitched closed. If more definition of the upper eyelid crease is required, the skin may be fixed to the deeper tissues with sutures.

COSMETIC SURGERY

Lower eyelid blepharoplasty

The main object of surgery to the lower eyelid is usually to remove fat, but if skin also needs to be removed, an incision is made just below the eyelid margin so that the skin can be lifted, either separately or together with the underlying muscle. The orbital septum and the three compartments of fat beneath it are exposed, and the excess fat is resected. Meticulous attention is paid to sealing the individual blood vessels before the excess skin is resected and the incision is closed. Excision of too much skin can lead to some of the potential complications of blepharoplasty (see below).

Sometimes lower eyelid surgery is done to remove fatty pouches that have developed in younger people as a family trait. As no skin needs to be resected in these cases, the fat can be removed through an incision made *inside* the lower eyelid, thus avoiding any visible external scarring.

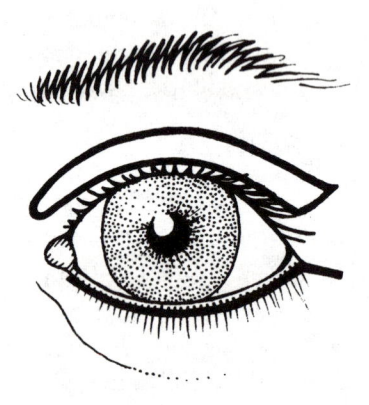

Blepharoplasty. Typical incision lines for upper and lower eyelid surgery.

After your operation

Whether or not you have to stay in hospital after your operation will depend on the extent of the surgery involved, on whether you have had a general or local anaesthetic, and on your surgeon's normal practice. Even if you have had a local anaesthetic, you will need someone to drive you home; you should not drive yourself until your eyes have stopped watering and your vision is completely clear. The amount of time you will need to take off work after your operation will depend on the extent of the surgery you have had.

If pads were placed over your eyes at the end of the operation, they will probably be removed within 12 hours. The stitches can be removed three to five days after surgery.

Pads soaked in cooled, boiled water may help reduce the swelling around your eyes. Bruising may persist for up to three weeks, and your eyes may continue to feel gritty and itchy for some time. No make-up should be used around the eyes for at least seven days after surgery.

The fine scars remaining once the wounds have healed will gradually fade and become less noticeable, and will probably be quite well hidden in the natural creases of skin around the eyes.

Possible complications

Complications of blepharoplasty include poor scar formation, hyperpigmentation, post-operative bleeding and haematoma (see p.97), damage to the inferior oblique muscle causing double vision, excessive fat removal, wound dehiscence (see p.99) following minor trauma and infection, inflammation of the eyelid margin, and eyelid laxity. The following are also possible.

Blindness
Although very rare after blepharoplasty, partial or complete blindness in one or both eyes can occur and is a risk that must

be considered before deciding to go ahead with surgery. Sometimes the cause of blindness may have been present but undetected pre-operatively. It is important to seek medical attention immediately if you experience increasing or continued pain, swelling or poor vision.

Watering of the eyes
Known as **epiphora**, watering of the eyes is common after eyelid surgery and is caused by blockage of the nasolacrimal ducts due to swelling. If it does not cease spontaneously, treatment may be required with antibiotic (or sometimes steroid) eyedrops.

Drooping of the upper eyelid
Although loss of sensation caused by damage to the nerves in the eyelid during surgery may continue for up to six weeks, it should still be possible to open and close the affected eye. Very occasionally, the muscle which opens the eye is damaged, causing permanent drooping (ptosis) of the eyelid, which will need to be surgically repaired.

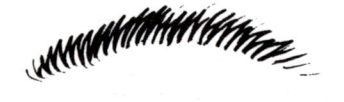

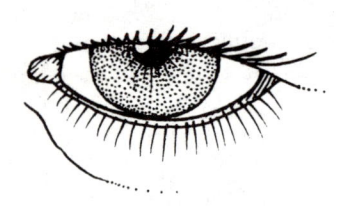

Ptosis of the upper eyelid.

THE EYES

Scleral show

Sometimes after lower eyelid surgery, an abnormal amount of the white of the eye (the **sclera**) becomes visible. This may be due to swelling causing partial paralysis of the muscle, in which case it is likely to improve as the swelling subsides and may respond to gentle massage. However, scleral show may be more difficult to resolve if it results from the removal of too much skin from the lower eyelid, excessive scarring of the underlying tissues, or an attempt at surgical correction that has pulled the eyelid down further. In these situations, it will always remain difficult to close the eye properly. Scleral show is more common in people whose lower lids have become weakened by age, smoking or the long-term use of contact lenses. It may also result from contracture of the scar under the skin.

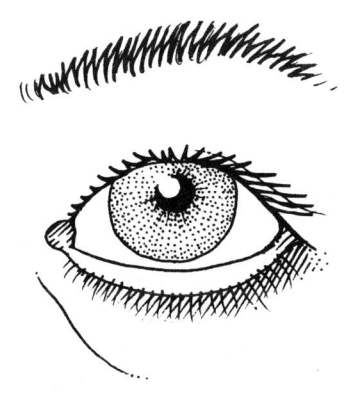

Sceral show.

Dry eye syndrome

As the scars in the eyelids heal and contract, the eyes may become dry. Artificial tears may be prescribed, and moist pads taped over the eyes at night can also help reduce swelling. The problem can be exacerbated in people who naturally produce very few tears, and is occasionally permanent.

Ectropion

Although similar to scleral show, ectropion is a more serious, functional, disorder in which the lower eyelid turns out, away from the eyeball. The eye becomes dry and irritated, and the condition will need to be corrected surgically.

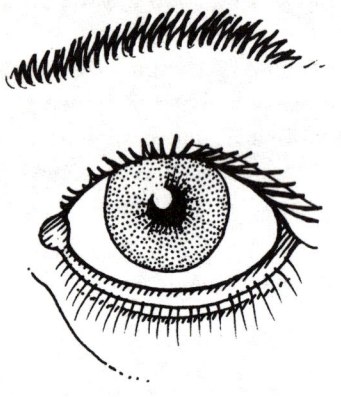

Ectropion with eversion of the lower eyelid.

Retrobulbar haematoma

Bleeding behind the eyeball following blepharoplasty is one of the few emergencies that can result from cosmetic surgery. Its cause is not known, but it may sometimes be due to excessive traction on a tissue when the fat is removed, although it can occur even when extreme care has been taken to avoid this.

The signs of retrobulbar haemorrhage include increasing pain in the eye, bulging of the eyeball (known as **proptosis**) and loss of the pupillary reflex followed by loss of vision. Urgent treatment is necessary as it can result in blindness in the affected eye.

CHAPTER 6

The nose

The size of the nose can be increased or decreased, bumps can be removed, and the shape of the nostrils can be altered by variations of an operation called **rhinoplasty**. However, there are limitations to how much tissue can be removed or added, and it is therefore important to discuss in detail with your surgeon exactly what it may be possible to achieve.

RHINOPLASTY

The width of the nose can be reduced by reshaping its bone and cartilage through incisions made inside the nostrils. If required, the length of the nose may also be reduced by the removal of some of the cartilage from its tip. Both operations are types of **reduction rhinoplasty** that are performed from *inside* the nose, leaving the external skin intact and therefore no visible scarring. Reduction of large nostrils is more difficult and does involve cutting the skin over the nose, with some degreee of scarring therefore being inevitable. The shape of a bent nose can also be improved by rhinoplasty, although it will not necessarily be possible to straighten it completely.

An operation known as **septoplasty** can be done to adjust the bone and cartilage which separate the two halves of the nose (the **nasal septum**) to straighten the nose or improve breathing.

Before your operation

At a pre-operative appointment, the surgeon will examine the inside and outside of your nose and may also take some photographs. Some surgeons use computer images to try to convey an idea of what the reshaped nose will look like, but these do not always give an accurate impression as it is not possible to predict the final appearance precisely. You should discuss with your surgeon exactly what your operation will involve and the possible results that may be achieved.

The surgeon will question you about your medical history and general health, and any necessary pre-operative tests will be arranged (see p.19).

The operations

Any type of rhinoplasty usually involves the use of a general anaesthetic and a night's stay in hospital post-operatively.

Internal (endonasal) rhinoplasty

An incision is made within each nostril, generally in line with its lateral wing (the **ala**) so that the skin and cartilage can be incised at the same time. The alar cartilage is dissected and reduced, and the dissection is continued along the top surface (dorsum) of the nose between the bone and muscles. The lateral alar cartilages are then separated from the central wall of the nose – usually keeping the mucosal lining of the nose intact – and are reduced using scissors or a knife.

The bony dorsal hump of the nose is reduced with a saw or an instrument called an **osteotome**. If only a small amount of bone needs to be removed, it may be possible to smooth it with a rasp. The nasal bone is then broken along its junction with the cheek to allow it to collapse inwards.

At the end of the operation, dressings may be placed inside the nostrils, and a plaster of Paris or plastic splint will be taped over the nose to hold the bones in place.

THE NOSE

Columella

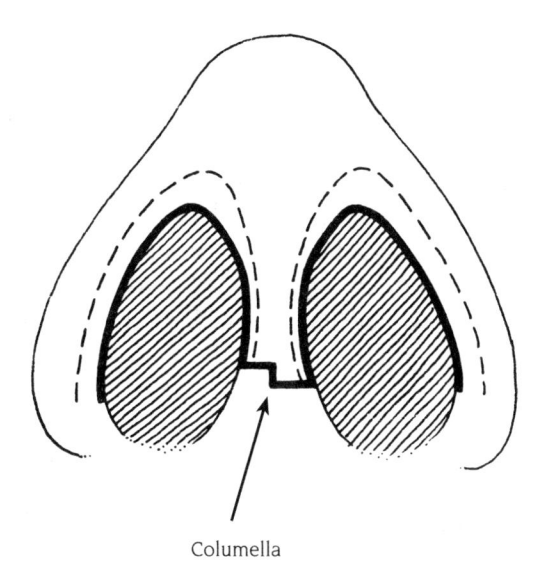

Rhinoplasty. The typical lines of incision that are made within the nostrils for internal (dashed line) and external (solid line) rhinoplasty. Note that for external rhinoplasty, the incision is continued externally across the columella.

External (open) rhinoplasty

The surgical procedure for external rhinoplasty is similar to that for the internal operation, except that the incision within each nostril is continued across the fleshy portion of the nasal septum, known as the **columella**. (A small external scar will therefore remain at this point.) The main advantage of external rhinoplasty is that the surgeon has a much better view of the entire nasal skeleton, particularly the tip area. It is therefore suitable for more complex operations or for secondary rhinoplasty to improve the results of previous surgery.

Once the incision has been made, the operation proceeds in a manner similar to that described above.

Tip surgery

Sometimes, all that is required is reduction of the tip of the nose, and in some cases this can be done on its own. However, if simply planing the cartilage is likely to result in an imbalance between the reshaped tip and the wider upper part of the nose, the nose may also need to be narrowed along its entire length by breaking the bone and pushing both sides inwards. The bone can either be broken from inside or by inserting a small chisel through tiny incisions made in the skin between the eyes and on the cheeks.

Apart from being used to reduce the tip of the nose, tip surgery can also be done to increase the height of a flat nose. If required, the nose can be reshaped with solid silicone, although it is more common in most countries to use a graft of the patient's own cartilage or bone.

After your operation

You may need to take mild painkillers for a day or two after your operation, and you will not be able to breathe through your nose until any dressings have been removed. The splint will probably be taken off after about seven days.

You should avoid sneezing or blowing your nose for a week or two, until the small wounds have healed. It may be advisable to sleep propped up for a few nights after any type of rhinoplasty to reduce swelling and aid easy breathing. A very blocked nose may be relieved by the gentle insertion of a cotton-wool bud dipped in hydrogen peroxide diluted with an equal volume of water, or by spraying the inside of the nose with a weak salt solution.

Although there is no medical reason why you should not be able to return to work almost immediately after your operation, you may not feel like doing so for a couple of weeks, by which time most of the bruising will probably have faded. It may be up to six months before all swelling has subsided and the full effects of surgery are apparent.

Possible complications

About 5 per cent of people who have undergone rhinoplasty have additional minor surgery because they are unhappy with the results – in some cases because irregularity of the dorsum of the nose has developed as new bone has formed during the healing process. Secondary rhinoplasty normally involves the removal of further small slivers of bone under local anaesthetic, but must be delayed for at least a year to allow time for the original scars to heal completely.

Most complications following rhinoplasty are minor and last only a few months. For example, some people suffer **rhinitis** (a constantly runny nose), which normally stops spontaneously within about six months. Any persistent swelling around the nose can usually be reduced by gentle massage. Repeated nose bleeds can occur post-operatively which, if they do not cease spontaneously, may be treated by cauterising the blood vessels responsible. Very rarely, obstruction of the nasal passages persists, resulting in an inability to breathe through the nose. Loss of sensation in the tip of the nose is usually temporary, although it can occasionally be permanent. Loss of the sense of taste is also sometimes reported.

The appearance of **spider veins** on the surface of the nose can be treated by injection (**sclerotherapy**), electrolysis or dye-laser.

CHAPTER 7

The lips

The lips tend to become thinner and longer with age, although thin lips can also be a natural feature in some younger people. Most cosmetic treatment for the lips is done to make them plumper, but there are also procedures to reduce thick lips or to change their shape to make them pout.

It should be noted, however, that most surgeons would not encourage the use of lip surgery, the results of which are variable and, when unsatisfactory, are difficult to correct. Probably the better option in most cases is temporary augmentation of the lips by means of injections. This chapter therefore gives only very brief details of the surgical and non-surgical techniques available.

COLLAGEN INJECTIONS

A relatively common, non-surgical procedure for augmenting the lips involves injecting collagen along their outer border. Collagen is present naturally in various tissues of the body, including the skin and bones, but the type used for cosmetic procedures is extracted from cowhide and purified to reduce the likelihood of it causing an allergic reaction (see below). Alternatives to collagen – but currently used less commonly – are fat and, more recently, hyalin, a natural substance present in the body which, for the purposes of cosmetic procedures, is derived from chickens.

Before the injections are administered, the lips are anaesthetised with anaesthetic cream. The injection itself also contains a local anaesthetic to help reduce the pain. Collagen injections are not always successful and need to be repeated regularly – usually every few months – as the collagen is gradually absorbed.

Possible complications

Collagen can give rise to an allergic reaction, causing red, itchy patches that may persist for several months and occasionally need to be treated with steroids. Surgeons therefore perform allergy tests before commencing collagen treatment, injecting a small amount of collagen into the arm and monitoring for any signs of an adverse reaction. However, these tests are not totally reliable as they can give false negative results. Allergic reactions, whatever their cause, can be so severe as to be fatal and, although this is a rare occurrence, it does need to be taken into account. Hyalin is apparently non-allergenic.

GORETEX

Goretex is most widely known for its waterproofing properties and its use in the manufacture of wet-weather clothes etc. However, it also has a cosmetic use, very small strips being threaded under the outer layer of the skin in the centre of each lip to plump it up. The results of this procedure are permanent.

Possible complications

The scars that form around the Goretex are sometimes so thick that the lips become hard. The Goretex may also move from the desired position under the skin. Although it does not cause allergic reactions, it can occasionally give rise to infection, requiring surgical removal, which is extremely difficult to accomplish without creating scarring.

SURGICAL TECHNIQUES

Grafting is a more permanent method of augmenting thin lips than any of the non-surgical procedures described above. It involves the removal of an elliptical portion of fat and dermis (the inner layer of the skin) from another part of the body, usually the abdomen or buttocks, which is then inserted into a hollow tunnel in the lip.

To alter the shape of the lips, a strip of skin is removed from the outer edge of each one. As the resulting wounds heal, the remaining skin contracts, causing the lips to pout. However, this operation usually leaves a visible scar and may result in the mouth being lopsided.

Thick lips can also be reduced surgically, by the removal of skin and fat from their inner surface.

Possible complications

Following any type of surgery, the lips will be swollen and bruised, possibly for several weeks. After grafting, most potential problems arise at the **donor site** from which the graft has been taken, which is likely to be quite painful for a few days until it heals. The surgeon will select a donor site where the small remaining scar will be as inconspicuous as possible. If a graft is rejected, it will have to be removed.

The results of the grafting of fat are unpredictable as there is almost always a significant amount of fat resorption. Therefore, this procedure often needs to be repeated to build up the desired amount of fat in the lips.

Infection is a common problem after lip surgery and requires treatment with antibiotics.

CHAPTER 8

The ears

Prominent ears – sometimes known as 'bat ears' – develop as a congenital 'abnormality' and can be corrected by an operation called **pinnaplasty** or **otoplasty**. Surgery may involve the construction of a fold in the cartilage that runs down the external part of the ear (the **pinna**) where this has failed to develop normally, or the removal of excess cartilage from this area.

In the UK, pinnaplasty is sometimes available under the NHS, particularly for children, and you may therefore wish to discuss this possibility with your family doctor before approaching a private surgeon.

PINNAPLASTY

For adults, the operation is normally a day-case procedure, involving the use of a local anaesthetic; general anaesthesia is used for children.

Before your operation

At a pre-operative appointment, the surgeon will examine your ears carefully and question you about your medical history and general health. Any necessary pre-operative tests will be arranged for you (see p.19).

The operation

Local anaesthetic and adrenaline (to reduce bleeding) are injected around and into the ears. To simulate a natural fold in

COSMETIC SURGERY

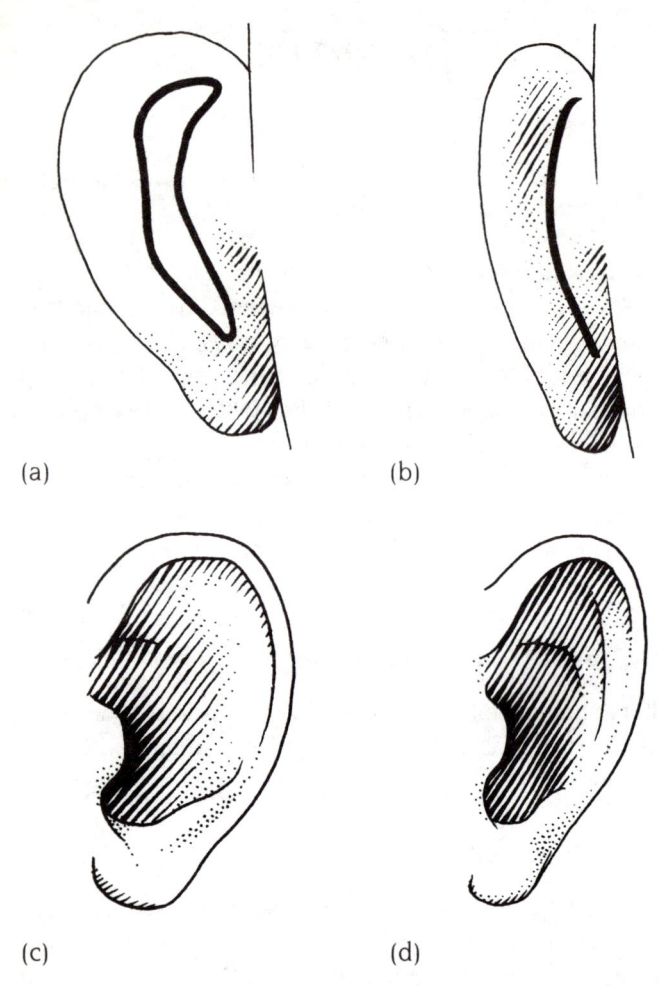

(a) (b)

(c) (d)

Pinnaplasty. (a) The lines of incision made at the back of the pinna to allow the cartilage to be folded. (b) The line of the resulting scar. (c) An example of an ear with no fold in the cartilage, viewed from the front, and (d) the same ear following surgery to create a fold in the cartilage and draw the ear inwards towards the head. The only visible scarring is at the back of the pinna.

the cartilage, an incision is made in the skin at the back of the ear once the anaesthetic has taken effect. The cartilage is then cut and reshaped to form a fold, sometimes with the aid of sutures, and the incision is closed with stitches. The procedure is repeated for the other ear before dressings are put in place. To remove excess cartilage from the pinna, a similar technique is used, with the exception that cartilage is excised rather than folded.

In both cases, the skin at the front of the ear remains intact, the post-operative scars being at the back of the pinna and relatively inconspicuous.

After your operation

Pinnaplasty is not normally very painful and most people do not require painkillers post-operatively. The dressings on the ears will probably be removed after about seven days, at which time the stitches may be taken out. As the ears can bleed quite profusely, care needs to be taken while the wounds are healing to protect them from knocks. Bruising and inflammation can persist for several days or weeks. A headband worn at night for two to four weeks keeps the ears flat during sleep. Very cold temperatures and excessive exercise can cause soreness following pinnaplasty and are best avoided.

Possible complications

Bleeding can be a problem after pinnaplasty, and sometimes leads to the development of haematomas (see p.97) that need to be removed surgically. Post-operative wound infection is not uncommon. Occasionally, the skin at the front of the pinna along the cartilage fold breaks down, although this usually heals spontaneously. Thick, keloid scars can build up once a wound has healed (see p.99).

COSMETIC SURGERY

Asymmetry of the two ears is quite common after pinnaplasty, which, although usually within normal limits, sometimes needs to be corrected by further surgery.

CHAPTER 9

The breasts

Surgery to reduce or augment the size of the breasts is known as **reduction** or **augmentation mammaplasty**, respectively. Whether you have large or small breasts depends to some extent on their normal growth (which is controlled by your genes), but also on hormonally controlled changes that occur during pregnancy and with age. As women get older, their breasts soften and droop as the glandular tissue within them gradually becomes replaced by fat. Drooping breasts can be lifted, and their shape restored, by an operation called **mastopexy** (see p.81).

Women have breast surgery for aesthetic reasons; to reduce physical symptoms caused by very large breasts; to reconstruct one or both breasts following **mastectomy**; or to correct noticeable asymmetry or, occasionally, the effects of congenital disorders such as **Poland's syndrome**, in which only one breast grows normally.

BREAST IMPLANTS

Various implants, of different shapes and sizes and made of different materials, are available for breast augmentation but all have a limited life expectancy. The look and feel of a breast implant will depend partly on the material it contains, which may be silicone, saline or oil. Each type of implant has inherent advantages and disadvantages and not all are appropriate for all women. Your surgeon will discuss any relevant restrictions with you when deciding on the most suitable type to use.

> **Silicone implants** Controversy arose concerning the use of silicone breast implants following claims of a link between the silicone gel they contain and the incidence of breast cancer and birth defects. There were also further claims of links with a range of autoimmune diseases such as rheumatoid arthritis, particularly following rupture of the implants in situ. It was suggested that leakage of silicone gel activates the body's defence mechanisms, instigating an autoimmune response and leading to self-destruction of cells and tissues. As a result, the use of silicone gel in cosmetic implants was banned in the USA in 1992, and superseded by the use of saline. However, these implants are still used in Britain and are currently in place in more than 100 000 women.
>
> Although the safety of silicone breast implants is constantly under review, recent reports have again raised questions about the potential problems that may be associated with implant rupture, and a new review is now likely to be commissioned by the government in Britain.
>
> If you are considering having silicone implants, your surgeon will discuss the possible problems with you, but do make sure that you raise any of your own concerns and that you fully understand the explanations you are given.
>
> It should be noted that this controversy only relates to the leakage of the *gel* form of silicone, which in its solid and oil forms still has a wide range of medical uses in most countries (including the USA), for example in joint replacement, in the shells of all breast implants and as a lubricant in syringes.

BREAST AUGMENTATION

Sometimes the breasts fail to grow (a condition known as **hypoplasia**) because of factors that have been present from birth or as a result of hormonal imbalance. Sometimes normal growth is restricted at puberty, or hormonal influences cause the breasts to become smaller after pregnancy. In addition to augmentation mammaplasty, mastopexy may also be undertaken to correct associated drooping of the breasts (see p.81).

Before your operation

At a pre-operative consultation, the surgeon will question you about your medical history and about your reasons for wanting breast augmentation. Your breasts will be examined, measured and felt for the presence of lumps, and you will be asked about any family history of breast cancer.

If you use an oral contraceptive pill, your risk of deep vein thrombosis following surgery may be increased (see p.101), and you may be told to stop taking it and use an alternative method of contraception for six weeks before your operation. You may also be told to avoid taking aspirin and similar drugs for at least two weeks pre-operatively as their blood-thinning properties may increase the risk of haematoma after surgery (see p.97). If you smoke, you should try to cut down, and should stop completely for at least three days before your operation (see p.96).

Breast implants are usually inserted through an incision made beneath the breasts, around the nipples or in the armpits, and the surgeon will discuss with you the most appropriate approach in your case, based on the following considerations.

An incision in the armpit leaves the least visible scar, but can make it more difficult to stop any internal bleeding that may occur during the operation and can cause damage to the nerves in the arm, leading to possibly permanent loss of sensation in the inner arm. An incision made around the pigmented areola that surrounds the nipple can reduce sensation in the nipple, limits access to the muscle of the breast, and leaves a visible scar. This type of incision is therefore only really suitable for the insertion of a small implant. An incision made beneath the breast allows the best access, and the original wound can be re-opened if a complication arises that requires further surgery, thus avoiding a second scar. However, in some cases the scar left by this type of incision is the most conspicuous.

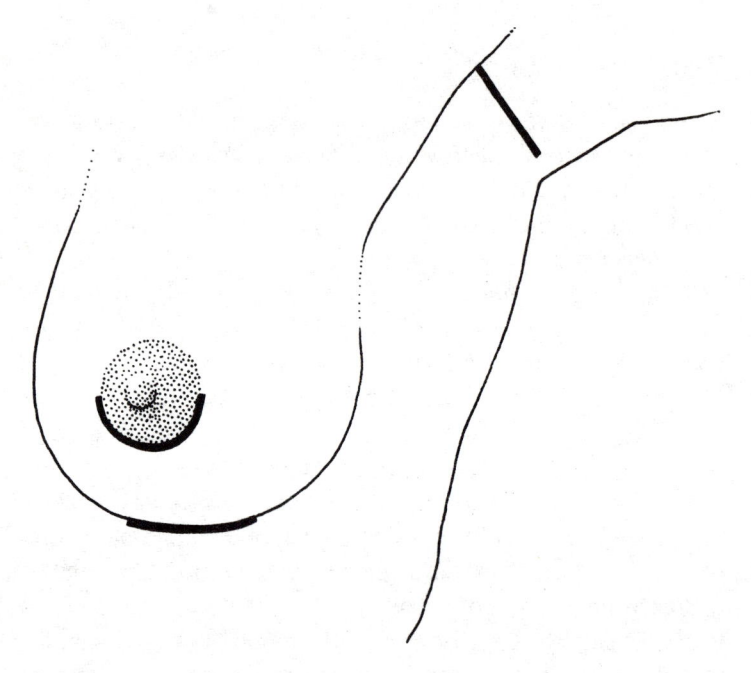

Breast augmentation. The dark lines indicate the different sites at which incisions may be made for the insertion of an implant.

The operation

Breast augmentation takes about an hour and a half to perform, and normally involves the use of a general anaesthetic.

Once an incision has been made at the chosen site, the implant is inserted either directly beneath the breast tissue or under the muscle behind the breast. The former may be appropriate for a droopy breast or for particular aesthetic reasons; the latter may reduce the risk of capsular contracture (see p.74), and the implant itself is less able to be felt when inserted in this position. When the implant is in place, the incision is closed with sutures.

Breast augmentation using a saline-filled implant can sometimes be performed endoscopically (see p.35), the shell of the implant being inserted through a small incision (about 2 cm wide) and filled once in place.

After the operation

You will probably have to stay in hospital at least overnight after your operation. Your breasts may be painful when you come round from the anaesthetic, and regular painkillers are usually needed for a couple of days. While in hospital, do ask for something stronger if necessary.

Drainage tubes may have been inserted near the implants to drain the blood and fluid which collect around them, and these will be removed once drainage reduces. The stitches will probably be taken out about seven to ten days after the operation, and a support bra should be worn both day and night for up to four weeks, during which time you should not sleep on your front – although it is likely to be too uncomfortable for you to want to do so anyway. Once the wounds have healed, the scars will gradually fade.

Driving will probably be possible about ten days after surgery, but it may be two or three weeks before you are fit to return to work. A full range of arm movements should be made several times a day, but all strenuous exercise, including swimming, should be avoided for about six weeks.

There is no reason why breastfeeding should not be possible after augmentation mammaplasty.

Possible complications

Some women are permanently unable to sleep on their front after breast augmentation, and some suffer pain, the cause of which cannot be determined. Sometimes implants have to be removed, together with the scar tissue that has formed around them, and as this usually leaves the breast flattened, most women prefer to have another implant inserted. Occasionally, an implant moves from its original position and surgery may be necessary to re-open the wound and reposition the implant.

The following specific complications can also occur.

Capsular contracture

The body reacts to any implant as 'foreign', and fibrous scar tissue forms around it – sometimes over a period of several years. This capsule of scar tissue may remain thin and pliable or, if the tissue shrinks and thickens, may compress the implant, causing it to become round and firm, which may cause tenderness. The shape of the breast may then alter and the implant may become hard. This process, known as capsular contracture, can occur at any time, although it is most common in the first year or two after surgery. Further surgery may be necessary to reshape the breast or remove the implant.

Wrinkling

Whatever the implant is made of, it will comprise a shell around a gel or fluid. It is possible for the outer shell to wrinkle, particularly if it contains saline or some other fluid, and this may be obvious if the breast tissue is thin. If required, a wrinkled implant can be removed and replaced by one of a different type. This problem is unlikely to occur with the more solid implant fillings such as 'cohesive gel'.

Rupture of the implant

Wear and tear or, more rarely, injury or a defect in the implant can cause its shell to rupture, enabling its contents (if fluid) to leak into the surrounding capsule. Increased scars and inflammation may result, and the implant may need to be removed surgically.

Although rupture of an implant does not necessarily cause any obvious signs or symptoms, you should seek medical attention if you develop pain or a change in the shape of a breast. Visualisation techniques such as magnetic resonance imaging, an ultrasound scan and/or mammography examination may be necessary to see if rupture has occurred.

Infection

Infection is a rare complication following breast augmentation, but may develop early or late – possibly months or years after surgery. When it does occur, the implant may have to be removed – at least temporarily. Infection can also weaken the skin and cause protrusion of an implant.

Change in nipple sensation

Although any change in nipple sensation after breast augmentation is unlikely to be permanent, the larger the implant the greater the risk. (Nipple sensation can occasionally be increased rather than decreased.)

Asymmetry

Lopsided implants can result in one breast being noticeably higher than the other. This type of asymmetry may occur because of a slight difference in the position of the implants or because of an inherent difference in the tissue and skin of the two breasts. Occasionally, it is due to an implant becoming displaced or to capsular contracture affecting one breast more than the other.

Thrombophlebitis

This problem may become apparent as localised pain, swelling and redness associated with inflammation of the superficial veins of the breast, and may respond to better breast support and anti-inflammatory drugs. However, as similar signs may occur as a result of infection, they should be reported to your doctor so that their cause can be determined.

BREAST REDUCTION

Breast reduction is not only sought for aesthetic reasons, but also to relieve symptoms related to enlargement of the breasts (known as **hyperplasia**), such as sweating and infection under the breasts, pain in the shoulders, neck or back, and discomfort in the chest.

Unusually large breasts may result from normal growth at puberty or from hormonal influences during pregnancy or the menopause. As breast size is determined by the amount of tissue rather than fat present in the breasts, dieting and weight loss tend to have little effect.

Reduction mammaplasty involves the removal of fat, glandular tissue and excess skin, as well as reshaping of the breasts and repositioning of the nipples. The extent of the pigmented areola around the nipple can also be reduced if required.

Before your operation

At a pre-operative appointment, the surgeon will take details of your medical history and question you about any members of your family who have had breast cancer. Your breasts will be examined and felt for the presence of any cysts or other benign or malignant lumps. It is important to have an approximate idea of the breast (cup) size you would like to have and to discuss this with your surgeon.

The operation inevitably leaves scars, usually in the shape of an inverted T, but the surgeon will explain to you any alternative sites of incision thought to be more appropriate.

Aspirin (and similar drugs) should be avoided for a couple of weeks pre-operatively as its blood-thinning properties can cause increased bleeding during and after surgery, which may increase the risk of haematoma development (see p.97). If you are a smoker, you should reduce the amount you smoke and stop

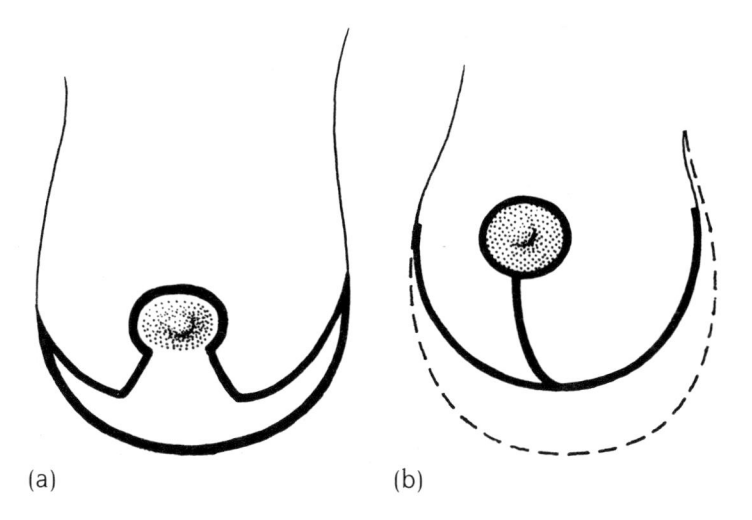

Breast reduction. (a) Typical lines of incision. (b) The solid lines show the positions of the scars following breast reduction. The shape of the original breast is indicated by the dashed line.

completely for at least three days before your operation (see p.96).

It is useful to take into hospital a bra that will provide good support after your operation. As your exact post-operative cup size cannot be predicted, it may be advisable to buy a couple of bras of different sizes at a shop that will accept the return of unworn goods. If this is not possible, you will probably be able to go out to buy a suitable bra two or three days after surgery.

The operation

Reduction mammaplasty usually takes about two to three hours and is carried out under a general anaesthetic.

The surgeon will measure your breasts and mark the proposed lines of incision. Precise surgical details will depend on the technique being used. In principle, excess skin and breast tissue is reduced and, as almost all hyperplastic breasts have ptosis, the nipples are elevated.

Once an incision has been made, a mound of breast tissue with the nipple still attached is separated from the underlying tissue, care being taken to avoid disrupting the blood and nerve supply to the nipple and remaining breast. The nipple is then moved up with the breast tissue to its new position. However, if your breasts are very large, it may be necessary to excise the nipple completely and graft it back into the required position.

The excess skin is excised and the remaining skin is stitched back into place before the procedure is repeated for the other breast.

After your operation

You may be in hospital for two or three days after a reduction mammaplasty. The dressing over your breasts will be removed after one to five days, after which you will need to wear a support bra, day and night, for about a month to support and help shape the breasts. The stitches will be taken out after about seven days.

The drainage tubes in your breasts will be removed as soon as blood and fluid loss reduces, usually within 24 to 48 hours. However, there will be quite extensive raw surfaces within the breasts, and leakage of fluid from the wounds or crusting around them may continue for a few days. Blood transfusion is only rarely necessary after reduction mammaplasty.

There is relatively little post-operative pain following this major operation, although regular painkillers are usually required for the first couple of days, and some discomfort may persist for several weeks. At the time of your first post-operative period, your breasts may swell and become quite tender and painful. Your breast shape will continue to improve over the next few weeks as the swelling subsides, and most signs of surgery will have faded by about 12 weeks post-operatively. As most of the scars will be under the folds of the breasts, they can be concealed by a bra.

You will need someone to look after you for a couple of days when you are discharged from hospital, and should not attempt to do heavy housework etc. for the first few days at least. You will probably be able to return to work after about two weeks, although you may continue to feel quite tired, with low energy levels, for several more. Sexual intercourse should be avoided for at least a week after surgery as arousal may cause the breasts to swell. Vigorous exercise should not be attempted for about six weeks.

Breastfeeding may not be possible after breast reduction, although this will depend on the type of surgery you have had.

The results of breast reduction are permanent, but gravity will continue to act.

Possible complications

Smoking and excessive body weight increase the risk of post-operative complications, and some surgeons will not agree to undertake reduction mammaplasty until these problems have been addressed.

Haematomas are not uncommon (see p.97), but usually resolve spontaneously, possibly with the discharge of a brown fluid from the wound. Occasionally, persistent haematomas have to be removed surgically.

Death of fatty tissue within the breast may lead to inflammation and a straw-coloured discharge. This is not normally a cause for concern, but may result in the development of lumps in the breast, which subside spontaneously in most cases.

Nipple loss
It is possible for the tissue of a nipple to die, partially or completely, the latter being an uncommon but serious complication of breast reduction. If complete nipple loss occurs, it is possible to reconstruct a nipple (and areola if required) from local breast skin or from a graft of skin taken from the upper, inner thigh. Nipple reconstruction is usually delayed until six months after the original operation, during which time an adhesive artificial nipple can be worn if desired.

Change in nipple sensation
Although some women experience increased nipple sensitivity after breast reduction, some loss of sensation can occur and may be permanent (see p.100).

Skin loss
It is quite common for the skin at the junction of the two scars on the breast to be slow to heal. Rarely, infection can lead to skin loss, which requires further surgery and results in increased scarring.

Abnormal scarring
Vertical scars can stretch, both in width and length, but they usually fade in time without the need for additional treatment, although they never disappear. However, pronounced scars can develop after breast reduction, usually under the breast, and the operation is therefore sometimes performed through a single vertical incision to reduce scarring.

Asymmetry
Occasionally, reduced and reshaped breasts are of different sizes or their nipples are in slightly different positions, usually as a result of pre-existing asymmetry that was not apparent pre-operatively. How noticeable this is will depend to some extent on the size of the breasts: a difference of 100 g between two large breasts will be less obvious than the same difference in small breasts.

BREAST LIFT

Sagging or drooping of the breasts can occur following childbirth or weight loss as the glandular tissue shrinks but the skin remains stretched. It is also a natural consequence of the effects of gravity with age. Mastopexy can be performed to reposition the nipples and lift the breasts without altering their size. It involves the use of a general anaesthetic, but is often done as day-case surgery (see p.21). If required, breast implants may be inserted at the same time, although some surgeons prefer to do this during a separate operation at a later date.

Women are usually advised to postpone mastopexy until they have completed their family, as pregnancy causes further sagging of the breasts.

The surgical procedure is similar to that for breast reduction (see p.77), but can sometimes be performed through a single incision made either vertically or around the areolar (circum-areolar). The nipple of each breast is repositioned (as described on p.78), the glandular tissue is pulled up through the incision, the excess skin is cut away, and the remaining skin is stitched back in place.

After surgery, the vertical scar in each breast may remain tight for some time, and the breast below the nipple may appear flat and square. It may be 12 weeks or more before the full effect of the operation becomes apparent. It is important to wear a bra which provides good support post-operatively.

The potential complications of mastopexy are similar to those following breast reduction (see p.79), although it is very rare to lose a nipple. The breasts are likely to droop again in time.

CHAPTER 10

Fat removal

There are various ways of removing fat from under the skin, but none of them is an alternative to losing weight by healthy eating and exercise, and all are unsuitable as treatments for obesity.

The surgical removal of fat from any site is called **lipectomy**, an example of which is the operation known as abdominoplasty (see p.86). However, with this exception, fat is more commonly removed by liposuction.

LIPOSUCTION

Liposuction is the most common of *all* operations performed in the USA. It involves the use of suction to remove fat deposits that remain despite attempts at losing weight, and results in a permanent change to the shape of the treated area, which will probably not be affected by any future changes in body weight. As fat is removed from quite deep beneath the skin, this is not an appropriate means of treating more superficial cellulite (see p.91).

As liposuction is only successful when the skin is sufficiently elastic to contract when the fat has been removed, it is only suitable for younger people, up to middle age. On the other hand, it is an unsuitable form of treatment for anyone not yet past their teens, during which body shape continues to change.

Liposuction can reduce fat deposits on the lower abdomen, hips, buttocks, outer thigh and inner part of the knee. The results on other parts of the body tend to be less successful. If required, it can be done at the same time as a face lift (to remove fat from under the chin, see p.41), with breast reduction (see p.76) or a tummy tuck (see p.86).

Sometimes ultrasound is used to turn the fat into oil before it is sucked out by the process of liposuction described below.

Before your operation

Pre-operative assessment is important. The surgeon will also examine you carefully to identify the area to be treated because the distribution of excess fatty tissue will alter when you are lying down on the operating table. You will be questioned about your medical history and general health, and any necessary pre-operative tests will be arranged (see p.19).

As use of a contraceptive pill may increase the post-operative risk of deep vein thrombosis (see p.101), women may be advised to use an alternative method of contraception for six weeks prior to surgery, particularly if the operation is likely to last longer than about 30 minutes.

The operation

Liposuction involves the use of a general anaesthetic or a local anaesthetic with sedation. It can be done either as day-case surgery or with an overnight stay in hospital post-operatively, depending on the volume of fat to be removed.

Tumescent liposuction is a variation of the technique of dry liposuction described below and involves injecting a mixture of saline, local anaesthetic, adrenaline (to reduce bleeding) and hyalase (a drug that enables the mixture to penetrate the fat deposits) into the operating site at the start of the operation.

The surgeon makes several small incisions (about 1 cm or less in length) around the areas to be treated and inserts a suction cannula (about 2–3 mm in diameter) through each one in turn. The cannula is tunnelled through the fat in various directions to loosen it, and a vacuum chamber attached to it then sucks the

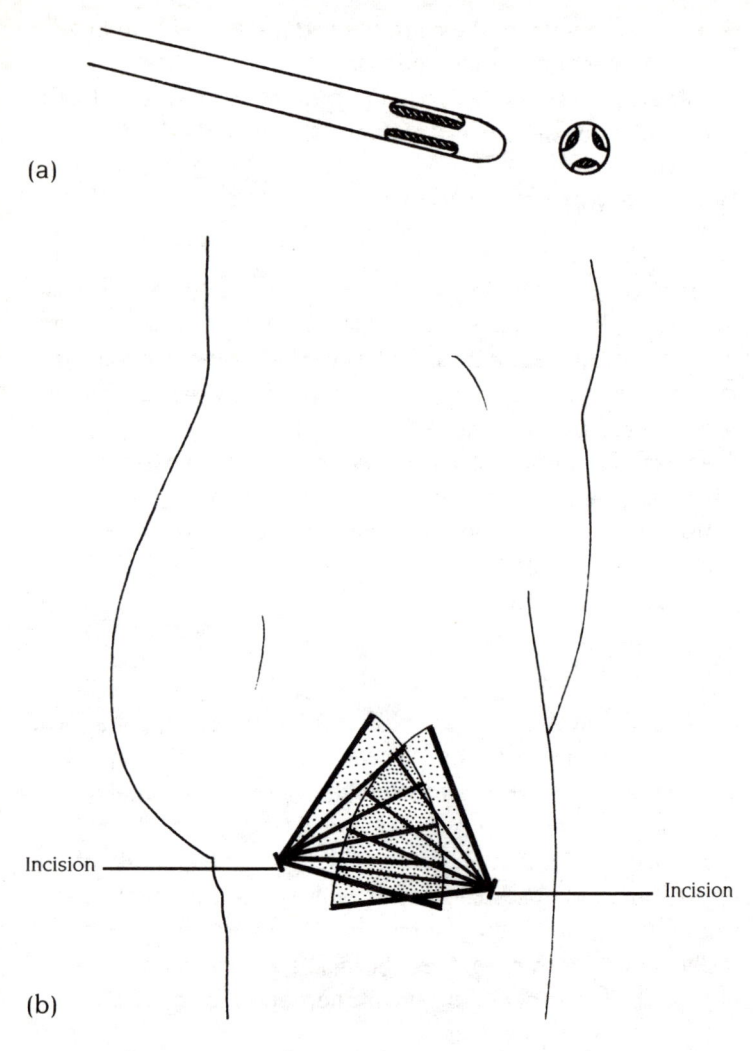

Liposuction. (a) A Mercedes cannula, a type often used to remove fat from under the skin. (The diagram of its cross-section explains its name.) (b) A cannula is inserted at various angles through small incisions to withdraw fat in a criss-cross pattern.

fat out. The process is repeated in a criss-cross pattern to reduce the risk of uneven fat reduction.

Once the surgeon is satisfied that an appropriate amount of fat has been removed and that your body contours are equal on both sides, the incisions are closed with one or two sutures and the area is strapped or covered with a pressure garment.

Occasionally, at the end of an operation in which large areas of the body have undergone liposuction, one or more drainage tubes may be placed underneath the skin to drain away the blood and fluid that collect there, and a drip may be inserted into a vein in an arm to replace the fluid lost from the body.

After your operation

If you have had only a small amount of fat removed, you should be able to leave hospital when you come round from the anaesthetic and feel able to do so. You may be given an elastic corset to wear for three or four weeks, which can be removed when you shower.

The treated areas may be very bruised and swollen, but you should not experience any real pain. Numbness caused by damage to the nerves may remain for several months, but sensation should return as the nerves regenerate. The effects of liposuction may not be fully apparent for about six months, until the swelling caused by fluid retention has subsided. Small scars will be apparent when the wounds have healed.

You will probably be able to return to work after anything from a few days to about three or four weeks, depending on the extent of the area treated.

Possible complications

Bruising may be quite severe after liposuction, and haematomas and seromas are not uncommon (see pp.97 and 99). Surface dimpling can develop if too much fat has been removed from just under the skin, if the skin is inelastic, or if excessive scarring forms beneath it.

Removal of large volumes of fat can cause the loss of significant amounts of blood, and blood transfusion is occasionally necessary. Even when blood loss is less substantial, anaemia can occur post-operatively, and iron tablets may have to be taken for a few weeks to correct it.

ABDOMINOPLASTY

The operation to remove fat and excess skin from the stomach is known as an **abdominoplasty**. Despite the somewhat trivial-sounding alternative name of 'tummy tuck', this is a major surgical procedure with significant potential complications (see p.90).

Abdominoplasty is sometimes performed at the same time as other abdominal surgery, such as hysterectomy, although any such combination would only be considered appropriate for a very healthy individual with no apparent contraindications.

Liposuction to remove excess fat from the abdomen (see p.82) cannot tighten the skin or muscles, and abdominoplasty may therefore be a more appropriate option when the skin has lost its elasticity and when the muscles of the lower abdomen need to be tightened.

The skin in the lower abdomen may become stretched for a variety of reasons. Following pregnancy – particularly multiple pregnancies – the skin and muscles of the abdominal wall stretch and a roll of fat may remain in this area despite dieting and exercise. Previous abdominal surgery resulting in multiple scars in the lower abdominal wall can also cause the skin to droop, and substantial weight loss can leave folds of skin over the abdomen.

Apart from the usual risk factors associated with surgery and the use of a general anaesthetic (see p.108), the main contraindications to abdominoplasty are obesity and smoking. Careful pre-operative assessment is necessary for anyone contemplating this operation.

Before your operation

At your pre-operative appointment, details will be taken of your medical history, you may be weighed, and the surgeon will examine your abdomen and note the presence of any existing scars. The amount of loose skin in the area will also be assessed; too little can result in increased post-operative scarring. You may be advised to do some exercises to strengthen your abdominal muscles before your operation.

The surgeon will also discuss with you the need for any additional treatment such as liposuction that can be undertaken at the same time as abdominoplasty.

You will be given subcutaneous heparin before your operation and TEDS to wear during it (see p.29) as this is a relatively lengthy procedure and you will be immobilised for a period afterwards – factors that can increase the risk of thrombosis (see p.101).

The operation

The operation will be done under a general anaesthetic and usually involves one or two nights in hospital post-operatively.

For a conventional abdominoplasty, an incision is made across the lowermost part of the abdomen, just above the pubic hair, extending laterally across the hips to just below the point of each hip bone. Sometimes, the line of incision may run above this level, depending on the patient's own choice and individual anatomy. A second incision is made in the skin around the **umbilicus**, which is separated on a stalk from the underlying tissue.

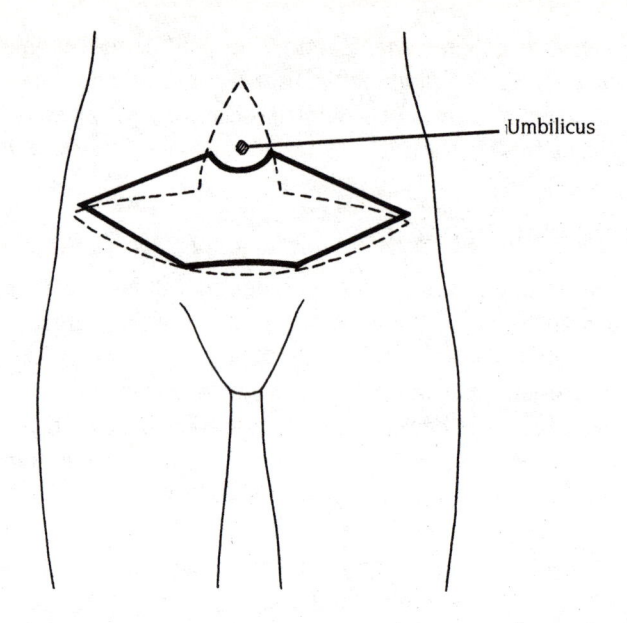

Abdominoplasty. Two of the alternative lines of incision that can be made, passing either above or below the umbilicus.

Different patterns of incisions may be used in specific circumstances, such as a fleur-de-lys pattern where a vertical incision is made in addition to the transverse one. In some cases, such as when the excess skin is in the centre or upper rather than lower part of the abdomen, the operation is performed through a single vertical incision.

The abdominal skin and fat are lifted off the underlying muscles, right up to the level of the lower ribs, and are tightened in a downward direction. Excess skin and fat are then removed.

Drainage tubes are inserted under the skin to remove the blood and fluid that collect there, and the skin incision is closed. The umbilicus is relocated into the appropriate position, and stitched in place.

Ocassionally a **divarication of the recti** needs to be corrected during abdominoplasty. Divarication can occur following pregnancy if a gap develops between the two vertical straps of rectus muscle which run down the abdomen on either side of the midline. The gap is reduced by tightening the muscle sheath with sutures.

The operation known as the **mini tummy tuck** is a variation of the technique described above in which the umbilicus is not relocated and is therefore in a slightly lower position than normal post-operatively.

After your operation

When you wake up from the anaesthetic, your legs will be bent, with your knees supported on pillows to help take some of the strain off the wounds. Your abdomen will be quite sore and you may feel sick and unable to eat or drink for at least the first post-operative day.

Once the drainage tubes have been removed, usually after 24 to 48 hours when blood and fluid loss has reduced, you will be able to get out of bed. It is important to become mobile as soon as possible after this operation to help reduce the risk of deep vein thrombosis (see p.101). If you cannot pass urine spontaneously, a urinary catheter will be inserted into your bladder to drain the urine from it.

Bruising may be quite extensive, but will gradually fade during the next few weeks. Once the stitches have been removed, about 12 days after surgery, you may be given a corset to wear for up to six weeks to apply pressure to the wounds as they heal. Although the scars will always be visible, the redness and swelling will continue to fade over a period of several months. If the scar around the umbilicus contracts, it may be difficult to keep this area clean.

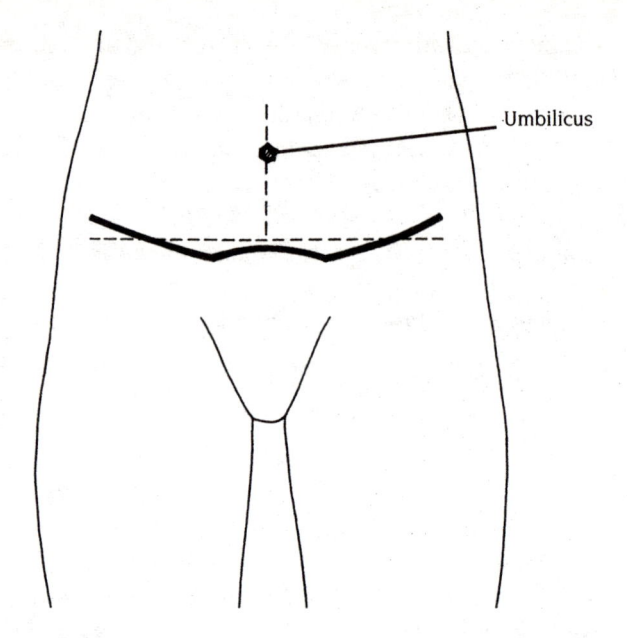

Abdominoplasty. Sites of the scars resulting from the alternative incisions shown in the diagram on p.88. Note that there is also a scar around the umbilicus.

Possible complications

Skin necrosis and wound dehiscence (see p.99) can occur after abdominoplasty, as can wound infection, haematomas and seromas (see pp.97–99). Sometimes fluid from a chronic seroma needs to be withdrawn with a needle. Pain, inflammation and swelling due to superficial infection of the skin around the wound (known as **cellulitis**) can be extensive. More major infection is rare, although **necrotising fasciitis** is slightly more likely to be associated with abdominoplasty than with other types of cosmetic operation (see p.98).

Deep vein thrombosis and pulmonary embolism are relatively

rare, but potentially very serious, complications and it is important to be aware of their symptoms and signs (see pp.101–102) and to seek medical advice if you are at all concerned.

Loss of sensation, which may occur below the navel and on the thigh, usually resolves in time, although occasionally damaged nerves fail to regenerate and numbness in the lower abdomen is permanent.

THE TREATMENT OF CELLULITE

Cellulite gives rise to an orange-peel appearance to the skin. It is most common in people who are overweight, although it can also develop in those who are underweight (but never in those who are undernourished). It has a tendency to occur in members of the same family, and cannot be cured by exercise. Cellulite may develop at puberty, during pregnancy and the menopause, and is under hormonal control. It can also occur in men with a high level of the female hormone oestrogen or with a low level of the male hormone testosterone.

There are various cellulite treatments available – including *mesotherapy*, *cellulolipolysis* and *superficial liposculpture* – many of which are not strictly surgical, and none of which is likely to be offered by an accredited plastic surgeon. Their effects are unproven and difficult to validate. The very fact that there are several such treatments may suggest that some – or all – of them do not work. It is therefore important to find out all you can about any cellulite treatment you are offered and about the experience of the person providing it.

PART III

General risks and complications of surgery

Some of the possible complications associated with any type of operation are relatively minor, but some are life threatening, and all should be considered by anyone contemplating cosmetic surgery.

It is important to be aware of the signs and symptoms of these complications so that medical attention can be sought when necessary and treatment can be given at an early stage, when it may prevent a more serious problem developing.

If you are at all concerned about anything that occurs once you have left hospital after your operation, do seek advice from your doctor or consultant surgeon.

CHAPTER 11

Possible post-operative complications

There are potential risks associated with any type of surgery, some of which cannot be anticipated or prevented but some of which may be reduced by taking some basic precautions. For example, the importance of finding an experienced and competent surgeon has already been discussed in Part I; by not doing so, you may be increasing the risks involved in your operation.

The risks of cosmetic operations performed by qualified, experienced surgeons and anaesthetists are quite small. Most post-operative complications are minor and resolve spontaneously, or with medical treatment, but some are more serious. Those associated with specific operations are dealt with in the relevant chapters, and the risks of general anaesthesia are discussed in Appendix I.

Your surgeon should explain all the possible complications to you, but do make sure you ask about anything you do not understand and do not be embarrassed to ask for something to be explained to you again if it is still not clear.

> **Obesity** Obesity adds to the risk of general anaesthesia. However, starting a long, strict diet before your operation may be inadvisable, and your surgeon will assess your weight at your pre-operative appointment, and will probably give you some guidance at that time. Some surgeons are reluctant to carry out any non-emergency operations on obese patients.

> **Smoking** Smoking increases the risks of specific complications of some cosmetic procedures for which tissue oxygenation is vital, such as abdominoplasty, breast reduction and face lift.
>
> If you are a heavy smoker and have not been able to cut down or stop altogether, you will be advised not to smoke in the days before your operation. It is, of course, much better to stop smoking some months before surgery. The carbon monoxide contained in cigarette smoke poisons the blood by replacing some of the oxygen that is carried in it and that is vital to processes such as wound healing. The nicotine in cigarettes reduces the blood supply by constricting the blood vessels. As for obesity, some surgeons may not wish to perform non-emergency operations on patients who smoke.

PYREXIA

Pyrexia is a raised temperature (fever), which often occurs in the first 24 hours after surgery, when it is usually of no significance. However, if persistent, its cause should be investigated as it can be a sign of infection or deep vein thrombosis (see p.101).

BRUISING

Bruising occurs as a result of blood escaping from blood vessels beneath the surface of the skin. It may not appear until several days after surgery and can sometimes be quite extensive, lasting for days or even weeks, although even severe bruising is rarely a cause for concern.

PAIN

The amount of pain experienced after any operation depends on the extent of the surgery involved as well as on the individual's own pain tolerance (see p.105). Although it is normal to feel some discomfort in a wound after an operation, it is unusual to have severe pain. Post-operative discomfort can normally be controlled by simple painkillers, but excessive pain can be a sign that an infection is developing. If you experience pain that fails to ease after a few days or increases at any time, you should seek medical attention.

BLEEDING

There is often a certain amount of oozing of blood or fluid from any wound, but this is unlikely to be heavy. If oozing persists, and particularly if it leaks from the wound dressing and soils your clothes, medical advice should be sought.

Very rarely, bleeding may continue and a wound may need to be explored at a second operation to tie off or cauterise a bleeding blood vessel that was not apparent during the original operation or that has started to bleed again post-operatively.

Haematoma

A haematoma is a blood-filled swelling that forms when a blood vessel continues to bleed or re-opens after surgery. It can also result from a disturbance of the normal blood-clotting mechanisms of the body. For example, people taking **anticoagulants** – drugs sometimes used to prevent blood clots forming – are more likely to bleed. There is also a variety of inherited bleeding disorders, such as haemophilia, which cause a similar disturbance of the blood-clotting mechanism, but these conditions should have been taken into account before any operation was considered.

Haematoma development is accompanied by pain, the formation of a hard swelling, and possibly a reddish purple discoloration in the skin. Bruising may appear around the wound or at some distance from it over the next few days. A raised temperature may develop if the haematoma becomes infected.

If you think a haematoma is forming, you should contact your family doctor or surgeon for advice. The blood is likely to be reabsorbed spontaneously within three or four weeks without the need for any treatment, but if heavy bleeding continues, with increased pain and swelling, you may need an operation to close off the blood vessel which is causing it. Your doctor may also wish to do specialised blood tests to check that your blood-clotting factors are normal.

WOUND INFECTION

Infection can sometimes occur in a wound following surgery. An infected wound will become red, hot to the touch, swollen and tender, and may be accompanied by a raised temperature. Pus or infected fluid may leak from it. Infection of this type may respond to simple cleansing of the wound, although antibiotics may be required.

If pus collects in an **abscess**, the wound will become red, hard and tender. The stitches may have to be removed to allow the pus to be released and a course of antibiotics may be necessary to prevent systemic infection.

Germs are likely to become concentrated around the stitches in a wound, and it is sometimes necessary for stitches to be removed to allow the resulting inflammation to resolve.

NECROTISING FASCIITIS

This is a very rare but potentially very serious bacterial infection that spreads rapidly near the surface of the body, destroying healthy connective tissue. Necrotising fasciitis can occur with any type of operation, although it is more often associated with abdominal surgery. Radical hospital treatment is required to remove the affected tissue surgically.

WOUND DEHISCENCE

Primary wound healing is important to limit scarring, but occasionally wounds fail to heal and may re-open – a process known as wound dehiscence. If dehiscence does occur, the wound may need to be resutured or covered with dressings until it heals.

SKIN NECROSIS

Skin necrosis is death of the skin, which can sometimes occur near a wound following surgery. If the affected area is small, the problem may resolve spontaneously without the need for treatment. A larger area of necrosis may require excision of the affected skin and possibly grafting; this problem is more common in the obese and in smokers.

FLUID COLLECTION

A skin flap may become raised by a collection of fluid that forms a **seroma** beneath it. The fluid is usually a light golden colour (not bloody) and probably comes from the lymphatics. It may have to be drawn off by inserting a needle into the scar – a procedure that may need to be repeated.

SCARRING

Scarring is inevitable after any type of surgical procedure and it is not always possible to predict how well a wound will heal and how much the scar will fade. A skilled surgeon will make sure that scars are as discrete as possible by making incisions in the lines of normal skin creases or within less conspicuous areas such as the hairline whenever practicable.

Some areas are prone to abnormal scarring, known as **keloid** scarring, especially the shoulder and chest. Further treatment may be necessary to settle the scar, and post-operative care of the wound may have to continue for several months to lessen the chance of a permanently obvious scar.

> **Caring for your scars** To assist in the healing of post-operative wounds and to help prevent contracture of scars, there are a few precautions that can be taken.
>
> Adhesive tape is kept in place over wounds for about two weeks to support the scars as they heal. When the tape has been removed, the scars should be massaged twice a day with an unperfumed cream such as E45 or Nivea. All scars should be protected from the sun with a total sunblock for at least a year as the skin will burn rather than tan. They should also be protected from chlorine, for example by being covered with a barrier cream during swimming in a chlorinated pool.

NERVE DAMAGE

The small nerves supplying the skin over the site of an operation are inevitably cut when an incision is made, occasionally causing an area around the wound to remain permanently numb. Although the size of the area of numbness will decrease with time, the sensation may never return completely. Many cosmetic operations carry the risk of injury to specific nerves, which is something you should discuss with your surgeon before going ahead with surgery.

Neuroma

Very rarely, small, painful, tender areas form in part of a scar, which may be due to a swelling of the cut nerve ends known as a neuroma. Nerve damage may lead to pain in the wound, which will be relieved temporarily by the injection of local anaesthetic. Continued pain may respond to steroid injection. Only rarely is surgery needed to remove a painful nodule.

Nerve palsy

Apart from causing loss of sensation, nerve damage can also result in loss of power known as palsy. This may last for days or months, but will eventually recover to a greater or lesser extent as the nerves regenerate. However, sometimes nerves never fully repair themselves, and loss of function of the affected part can result.

CHEST INFECTION

Chest infection is possible after general anaesthesia for any type of operation, particularly if a painful wound makes breathing difficult. It is more common amongst smokers and when mobility is restricted post-operatively. It is important to keep the lungs well aerated after surgery and you may be shown how to do some deep-breathing exercises before you leave hospital, although this is rarely necessary following most cosmetic operations.

DEEP VEIN THROMBOSIS

The normal activity of the muscles in the legs helps to keep the blood moving through them, but during long periods of bed rest or anaesthesia, these muscles are inactive and the circulation of blood in the legs slows down. This may lead to coagulation of the blood within a blood vessel (known as **thrombosis**) and formation of a blood clot (**thrombus**), which may block the passage of blood through the vessel.

If a blood clot forms, treatment with anticoagulant drugs will be necessary to reduce the risk of pulmonary embolism (see below). High-dose heparin is given initially, followed by warfarin for several months to thin the blood and help prevent it clotting.

If your mobility is likely to be restricted post-operatively, you may be given anti-embolism stockings to wear during and after your operation until you are mobile again (see p.29). These stockings are thought to help reduce the risk of blood clots forming by exerting a graded pressure along the length of the leg to assist the circulation of blood through it. Raising your legs when sitting will also help to reduce the risk of thrombosis. If you are thought to be at particular risk of thrombosis, you may also be given a course of injections of low-dose heparin until you are mobile again.

Medical advice should be sought *immediately* if you experience pain, swelling or inflammation, particularly in the calf of a leg, as these may be signs of thrombosis.

PULMONARY EMBOLISM

The most serious risk associated with thrombosis is that if a piece of a blood clot breaks off, it forms an **embolus** that can travel through the circulation and lodge in the lung, causing pulmonary embolism. Pulmonary embolism can be life threatening and requires urgent treatment, and therefore the cause of any pain in the chest after an operation must be investigated immediately.

APPENDICES

APPENDIX 1

Anaesthesia and pain relief

Anaesthesia is an important part of any operation. Local anaesthetics, often administered by the surgeon, are relatively straightforward, but a general anaesthetic must be administered by a trained anaesthetist, who will remain with you throughout your operation.

Most people undergoing surgery are concerned about the amount of pain or discomfort they will experience. This varies from person to person, and of course depends on the extent of the surgery involved. After the more major operations, some people have only slight discomfort for 12 to 24 hours, whereas others may need pain-killing injections for a day or two. While in hospital, do make sure that you let a nurse or doctor know if your pain is not being adequately controlled as it may be possible for you to be given something stronger. Any analgesics that you need once at home should be taken regularly to be effective.

LOCAL ANAESTHESIA

A local anaesthetic is a drug that blocks the sensation of pain in the area of the body into which it is injected. It does not put you to sleep and has the advantage of allowing you to be able to get up and move around immediately after surgery. Local anaesthetics do not cause post-operative nausea or drowsiness and there is very little risk involved in their use. The anaesthetic may sting as it enters your body, and some people find the injection painful. Although you are likely to be able to sense touch once the anaesthetic has taken effect, you should say if you feel any pain as you may require an additional injection.

Nerve block

A nerve block involves the injection of local anaesthetic around specific nerves, possibly a short distance from the site of the operation. Nerves follow a predictable path through the body and there are several sites at which they can be conveniently anaesthetised.

GENERAL ANAESTHESIA

A general anaesthetic will put you to sleep so that you have no feeling in any part of your body. It may be an **intravenous anaesthetic**, injected into a vein in your hand or arm through a plastic tube, or an **inhalational anaesthetic** in the form of a gas that you breathe in. In fact, both types are normally used, although you will probably only be aware of the injection that sends you off to sleep. The advantages of general anaesthesia are that you will be in a deep sleep throughout the operation and will not move or otherwise interrupt the work of the surgeon, and that you will be unaware of the surgery taking place.

Before your operation

When you are taken from the ward, you may go first to the anaesthetic room or straight to the operating theatre to be given your anaesthetic. The anaesthetist or ODA (see p.34) will fit some monitoring devices to watch over you while you are asleep. These may include a little probe which goes on your finger to measure the amount of oxygen in your blood, an electrocardiogram to monitor your heart, and a cuff around your arm to measure your blood pressure. Once the anaesthetist is happy with the readings from these monitors, your anaesthesia will start. During your operation, the anaesthetist will make sure that you remain asleep and that the function of your heart and lungs is satisfactory.

Once the anaesthetic has been injected into the tube in your hand or arm, you will fall asleep within seconds. The drug that makes you go to sleep may sting a little as it enters the vein from the cannula, but this feeling does not last long.

Several different types of drugs will be given to you during your operation, which may include:

* *induction agents* to bring on sleep;
* *maintenance agents* to keep you asleep;
* *analgesics* to stop you feeling pain after the operation;
* *anti-emetics* to help stop you feeling sick after the operation.
* *muscle relaxants*.

Local anaesthetic is often injected into the wound during surgery to reduce the pain when you wake up.

When the operation is over, the anaesthetist will stop giving you the drugs that were keeping you asleep, and you will be taken to a recovery room.

The recovery room

You will stay in the recovery room, with your vital functions still being monitored, until you are fully awake and ready to be returned to your own ward.

If you are in any pain when you wake up, the staff in the recovery room will be able to give you something to relieve it, probably an injection through the cannula that was used to put you to sleep or into your arm or leg.

The step-down ward

If you are having day-case surgery, you may be taken from the recovery room to a step-down ward where the nurses will make sure that you are fit to go home and that your journey will be safe and pain free. Nursing staff will also want to be sure that you have a responsible adult to care for you once you are at home.

Back on the ward

If you are not going home the same day, you will be taken back to your own ward or private room, where the anaesthetist may visit you to ensure that you are having adequate pain relief and have no ill-effects from your operation. Do tell the anaesthetist if you have any concerns or questions.

SIDE-EFFECTS OF GENERAL ANAESTHESIA

There are side-effects related to the use of general anaesthetics, but these are usually minor and do not last very long. The most common are nausea and vomiting. You may also have a sore throat, possibly due to the 'dry' anaesthetic gases used to keep you asleep during surgery, or to the tube that may have been placed in your throat to maintain an airway and help you to breathe. Whatever the reason, any soreness usually disappears after two or three days and can be eased by simple painkillers. The muscle relaxants sometimes used during anaesthesia can cause muscle aches and pains, which should improve within about 48 hours.

RISKS OF GENERAL ANAESTHESIA

People with certain medical conditions, such as serious heart or lung disease, may not be given general anaesthetics as they are potentially at greater risk.

Some people are afraid of being put to sleep by a general anaesthetic, but the risk is small. Advances in anaesthesia over recent years have been tremendous. Although complications still occasionally occur and, very rarely, people do suffer brain damage or even die during surgery – risks that need to be borne in mind – you are far more likely to be killed in a road accident than to suffer any permanent ill-effect from the use of an anaesthetic. However, if you are worried about the risks involved, do discuss them with the surgeon or anaesthetist.

PATIENT-CONTROLLED ANALGESIA

In some hospitals, patient-controlled analgesia (PCA) may be offered after the more major operations such as breast surgery and abdominoplasty. The PCA technique allows patients themselves to control the amount of analgesic they receive, and is generally a better way of providing pain relief than most of the conventional forms.

If a PCA machine is available, you will be given clear instructions about how to use it. It is basically a pump that delivers a pain-killing drug into your body each time you press a button. It is programmed to allow you only a safe limit of the drug, which is usually delivered via a cannula in a vein in your hand or arm. When you press the button, your pain should start to reduce within five to ten minutes. If it does not do so, press the button again. As the machine has a built-in safety control to prevent you receiving too much of the drug, you can press the button as often as you like. However, it is important that you do not let anyone else use your machine as doing so would remove the safety feature. If, despite pressing the button several times, your pain is not being relieved, tell a nurse or doctor as it may be possible for the machine to be reset to deliver a stronger dose of the drug.

The counter on your PCA machine will be inspected at regular intervals to see how many times you have pressed the button and how much analgesic drug you have received. Once it is clear that you are reducing the amount of drug you need, and therefore your pain is improving, the machine setting will be changed to deliver a lower dose at each press of the button. Patient-controlled analgesia (or analgesic injections) can normally be replaced by analgesic tablets after 24 to 48 hours.

APPENDIX II

Paying for your operation

Most cosmetic surgery is done at private hospitals or cosmetic clinics or, in the UK, in the private wards of NHS hospitals.

PRIVATE HEALTH INSURANCE

If your operation can be classified as medically necessary, and you have private health insurance – either through the company for which you work or that you pay for yourself – your policy may cover you for the costs involved. However, these cases are relatively uncommon and this section therefore gives only general details of what to do if you have private health insurance. Your Company Secretary or health insurance company should be able to answer any specific queries you have.

It is always worth checking with your insurance company exactly what is covered by your particular policy, and asking for *written* confirmation. Do not be afraid to keep asking questions until you are certain you know exactly which costs you will be responsible for paying yourself. For example, does your insurance cover all follow-up appointments? Some health insurance policies have an annual maximum pay-out, so if you have recently had any out-patient investigations or treatment, you should make sure you have not already reached your limit. Most private hospitals have an administration officer who will check your insurance policy for you if you are in any doubt and will try to sort out any problems you have.

Do read your policy carefully, and any information sent to you by the hospital, as unexpected charges, such as consultants' fees that may not be covered, could add up to quite a lot of money. Some insurance policies have a ceiling cost for consultants' fees and, if the fees quoted by your consultant exceed this limit, you will have to pay the extra yourself.

Some types of private health insurance require a form to be filled in by a family doctor to confirm that the operation is necessary and cannot be done in an NHS hospital within a certain time period. A small fee is payable to the doctor for this service, which is not redeemable from the insurers.

If your operation is being paid for by insurance, you will be asked to take a completed insurance form with you when you are admitted to hospital. You should have been given some of these forms when you first took out your policy, but your insurance company will be able to supply the correct one if you have any problems. If you are covered by company insurance, the form will probably be filled in and given to you by your Company Secretary.

After you are discharged from hospital, you may receive accounts from the surgeon and anaesthetist. These should either be sent to the hospital, for forwarding to your insurance company with the hospital account, or direct to your insurer. If you send the accounts to your insurer, make sure you quote your policy number and the date and place of your operation in case the insurance company has not yet received the hospital account and has no record of your operation. Always take, and keep, a copy of all accounts and completed claim forms.

PAYING FOR YOUR OPERATION YOURSELF

If you are paying to have your operation done privately, which is most likely to be the case, your surgeon should be able to tell you how much it will cost. Alternatively, the Bookings Manager at the private hospital or cosmetic clinic where your operation is to be carried out will let you have a written quotation of the costs involved.

Fixed Price Care

Many private hospitals have a service known as Fixed Price Care: a price can be quoted to you before you enter hospital that covers your operation and a variety of other hospitalisation costs. However, at some hospitals, the fixed price only includes hospital-related costs such as accommodation, nursing, meals, drugs, dressings, operating theatre fees, X-rays etc.; at others, the consultants' fees are also included. Make sure you obtain a note of everything included in the quotation *in writing before* you enter hospital.

The price you are quoted may or may not include any treatment required should some complication arise that is related to your original operation and that necessitates you having to remain in hospital longer than expected or be re-admitted within a limited period of time after your discharge. You should also ask your consultant whether his or her quoted fees (and those of the anaesthetist) would include such an eventuality.

Settling your bill

The only other payments you will have to make to the hospital before you are discharged will be for telephone calls, any alcohol you have with your meals, food provided for your visitors, personal laundry done by the hospital, and any similar items that you would have to pay for in a hotel. Visitors can usually eat meals with patients in their rooms, and tea and snacks can be ordered for visitors during the day. (You will also have to pay these extra charges before you leave the hospital if you are being treated under private health insurance.)

Case histories

Major problems following cosmetic surgery are relatively uncommon, although that is not the impression one might obtain from the media, which tends inevitably to highlight the more newsworthy complications that can occur.

The case histories in this section are not intended to make any specific points, but some of them help to illustrate the more common minor post-operative complications that usually resolve spontaneously or with medical intervention.

The people whose experiences of cosmetic surgery are briefly described have been chosen at random; it is only by chance that they are all women. All the operations were done at private hospitals and all were performed by surgeons who also work for the NHS.

CASE 1

Amanda is 51. Having wanted to have the hump removed from her nose and her nostrils made symmetrical for as long as she can remember, she had been deterred by the cost and a reluctance to appear vain. However, after inheriting some money, she made enquiries at several cosmetic clinics, eventually being referred by her family doctor to a plastic surgeon with a private practice.

Although the surgeon explained to Amanda that it would not be possible to make any drastic alterations to the shape of her nose, as doing so would upset the balance of her facial features, she decided to go ahead with rhinoplasty.

Amanda stayed in hospital for one night post-operatively. She found being unable to breathe through her nose after the operation quite frightening – particularly as she is asthmatic – but the problem improved when the packing was removed from her nose before she left hospital. The plasters across her nose and forehead irritated her skin until they were removed by the surgeon after about ten days, and she stayed at home during this time as she was embarrassed by her appearance. However, she was pleased not to have any visible stitches or wounds – the operation having been performed endonasally. The swelling and bruising gradually faded over the next few weeks.

Although Amanda found the whole experience quite unpleasant, she is quite happy with the results, but does feel that she would have benefited more if she had had the operation at a younger age.

CASE 2

Deborah is 29, 5 feet 1 inch tall, and weighs 7 stone. She had contemplated breast reduction surgery for several years, her size 32GG bust having caused her to develop rounded shoulders and backache problems since the age of 16. She had always found it difficult to buy clothes to fit – ready-made dresses were never an option with her size 8 lower body and size 14 upper body.

Deborah eventually telephoned her local NHS hospital to ask for the names of some suitably qualified and experienced plastic surgeons with private practices, and her family doctor wrote to the surgeon she selected to request an appointment for her.

Deborah stayed in hospital for two nights post-operatively; the only real pain she experienced during this time being when the two drains in each breast were removed. However, once at home, when the effects of the anaesthetic had worn off, her breasts became quite painful and she found it difficult to get comfortable and to sleep at night. The pain gradually reduced over the next few days, although the bruising, swelling and tenderness remained for some time.

Deborah took things very easily until ten days after her operation when the stitches were removed and the wounds were covered with adhesive tape. She wore a firm-control bra during the day for several weeks, and a maternity bra at night, having found this provided the small amount of support she needed but was a bit more comfortable than the 'sleep bra' that had been recommended.

Although the wounds in one breast healed well, the scars being pale and barely visible after a year, the scars on the other breast remained thick and purple, and Deborah's surgeon covered them with adhesive tape and advised her to massage them.

Deborah had not wanted a drastic reduction in her breast size, and is very pleased with the results of her operation and her 32D bust. She only regrets that she did not have it done earlier.

CASE 3

Frances is 29. When her name was first added to an NHS waiting list for reduction mammaplasty, she had a bust size of 38G and had been suffering shoulder pain for some time. However, while waiting for an operation, she lost a substantial amount of weight, her bust size changed to 34G, and she decided to have the operation done privately as soon as possible.

Frances stayed in hospital for two days after her operation and was warned to take things easy for a week or so when she went home. Although she did have some post-operative pain, it eased once the stitches had been removed after about two weeks. She returned to work four weeks after surgery but, finding it difficult to manage, she stayed at home for a further two weeks.

The quite extensive bruising gradually faded, as did the vertical scar on each breast, and at her six-month follow-up appointment all was pronounced well. However, a couple of weeks later

Frances developed a cyst in one breast, and was referred back to the surgeon by her family doctor. Fluid was withdrawn from the cyst with a needle and Frances started a course of antibiotics. Unfortunately, as soon as she came to the end of the course, another cyst developed in the other breast – a pattern that was to be repeated several times during the next five months, each cyst being aspirated by the surgeon as it developed. There was no obvious cause for this problem, and Frances was advised to take multi-vitamin tablets and evening primrose oil until the cysts stopped developing, which they eventually did.

Despite these problems, Frances is very pleased with the results of her operation and her size 34C bust.

CASE 4

Sally is 28. She has always had small breasts, but after losing a lot of weight following the births of her two children, her bust size reduced to 32AA. Although normally quite self-confident, she began to feel unfeminine and to wear baggy tops to hide her flat chest. Sally finally discussed breast augmentation with her family doctor, who requested an appointment for her with an NHS surgeon. When an operation proved to be unavailable under the NHS in her area, she made an appointment with a private plastic surgeon who had been recommended by a friend.

Sally stayed in hospital for one night post-operatively, during which time her breasts were quite painful. She was advised to rest for a week and had help at home for a few days.

A year later, the scars on Sally's breasts are barely visible and she is very pleased with her size 34B/C bust.

CASE 5

Kate is 36. Having had two children, and having lost a substantial amount of weight over the years, she decided to undergo mastopexy to reshape her breasts and tighten the loose skin. Her family doctor recommended a surgeon with a private practice at a local hospital and, although somewhat daunted by the surgeon's explanation of the operation and its potential risks, she decided to go ahead.

Kate stayed in hospital for two nights post-operatively as her breasts were very swollen. When she did go home, she found the 20-minute drive from the hospital made her very sore. A few days later, a yellowish discharge began to leak from the wound in one breast, and each time Kate changed the dressing the surface of the wound re-opened. After a week, she went to her family doctor, who sent swabs of the discharge for analysis and started Kate on a course of antibiotics. Kate continued to bathe the wounds with salt water several times a day for a couple of weeks, until the infection had cleared and they finally healed.

The swelling and tenderness in her breasts continued for about four or five weeks, and some bruising remained for a couple of months. Kate was able to drive about four weeks after her operation, but continued to find it too uncomfortable to wear a seatbelt for a further four weeks. She was off work for two months.

Four months after surgery, the scars on the breast which had become infected are still quite obvious, whereas those on the unaffected breast are fading. Kate has a small lump on the previously infected breast, which is thought to be a blocked vein that may resolve spontaneously in time.

Kate is pleased with the outcome of her operation and is optimistic that all her scars will eventually fade.

CASE 6

Leoni is 18. She has always had 'bags' under her eyes, and a couple of years ago made an appointment with a plastic surgeon (chosen from a list given to her by her family doctor) to discuss lower eyelid blepharoplasty. Because Leoni's mother was concerned about the use of general anaesthesia, the surgeon agreed to perform the operation using a local anaesthetic.

Leoni's operation lasted just under an hour, her lower eyelids being anesthetised with several injections into her mouth and cheeks and anaesthetic drops in her eyes, all of which she found quite unpleasant. Her lower eyelids were quite sore after the operation, and her eyes watered and her vision was blurred for a few hours, during which time she found it difficult to focus. However, she did not need to use painkillers once she had left hospital the following day.

Leoni used the herbal remedy arnica and the quite extensive bruising around her eyes had faded considerably within about five days. She also massaged the skin around her eyes every day, and most of the swelling had subsided by the time she returned to work two weeks after her operation.

Three months later, Leoni is quite pleased with the results of surgery, although the improvement is not as marked as she had hoped it would be. However, she is expecting the remaining swelling to continue to subside and the full effects of her operation to become apparent in time.

Medical terms

Abdomen The body cavity between the diaphragm and the floor of the pelvis that contains the organs of digestion – the stomach and intestines.

Abdominoplasty An operation to remove fatty tissue and excess skin from the abdomen and to reposition the umbilicus.

Abscess A collection of pus secondary to localised infection.

Ala (of the nose) The wing of the nostril that is supported by cartilage.

Alar cartilage The cartilage supporting the wing of the nostril.

Allergy An abnormal reaction to a substance. An allergic reaction can be mild, causing an itchy rash, or severe, leading to fainting, vomiting, loss of consciousness or death.

Anaemia A condition caused by deficiency of red cells or haemoglobin in the blood.

Anaesthesia The absence of sensation.

Anaesthetic A drug which causes loss of sensation in part or all of the body.

Anaesthetist A doctor trained in the administration of anaesthetics.

Analgesic A drug that blocks the sensation of pain; a painkiller.

Antibiotic A substance that kills bacteria or prevents them replicating.

Anticoagulant A substance that thins the blood and prevents it from clotting.

Anti-embolism stockings Stockings sometimes worn during an operation and any period of immobilisation post-operatively.

The stockings assist the circulation of blood in the legs and may help prevent blood clots forming.

Anti-emetic   A drug that helps to reduce feelings of sickness.

Areola   The pigmented part of the breast.

Axilla   The armpit.

BAAPS   British Association of Aesthetic Plastic Surgeons.

BAPS   British Association of Plastic Surgeons.

Blepharoplasty   Surgery to remove excess skin and/or fat from the upper or lower eyelids.

Blood transfusion   The transfer of blood from one individual (the donor) to another (the recipient) that is sometimes necessary after surgery when substantial volumes of blood have been lost. Blood from the patient is cross-matched pre-operatively to make sure that blood of the same type is transfused. The transfusion of incompatible blood can lead to serious complications.

Breast augmentation   Surgery to increase the size of the breasts by the insertion of implants.

Breast reduction   Surgery to remove fat, glandular tissue and excess skin from the breasts to reshape them. It also involves repositioning of the nipples.

Brow lift   An operation to cut the muscles that lower the eyebrows.

Cannula   A very fine tube or needle, usually made of plastic. Fluids can be introduced into or removed from the body through an intravenous cannula inserted into a vein, usually in the back of the hand. Intravenous cannulas are also used to administer anaesthetic drugs during surgery.

Capsular contracture   Tightening of the capsule of fibrous scar tissue that forms around a foreign body such as a breast implant. The breast becomes firm to the touch or, in severe cases, hard and painful, and the implant may have to be removed.

Cardiovascular   Relating to the heart and blood vessels.

Cartilage   A specialised body tissue that is firm but flexible.

Catheter A thin tube used to withdraw fluid from or introduce it into the body.

Cauterise To burn a part with heat or some other agent. During surgery, bleeding from the severed ends of small blood vessels is stopped by sealing them with the tip of an instrument heated by an electric current.

Cellulite Dimpled skin with an orange-peel appearance, the production of which is hormonally controlled and occurs during puberty, pregnancy and the menopause.

Cellulitis Inflammation of connective tissue that can occur around a wound.

Cellulolipolysis Electrical treatment sometimes used for cellulite. An electric current is administered to the fat cells beneath the surface of the skin via pairs of fine needles. The current alters the electrical charge of the fat cells, which then burn up energy as they attempt to restore their natural state.

Chemical peel The use of corrosive chemicals to remove the outer layer of skin and erase fine lines, scars and other superficial blemishes.

Collagen Proteins which occur in bone, cartilage and connective tissue. Purified collagen extracted from cowhide can be injected into the lips to plump them up.

Columella The fleshy part of the nasal septum that divides the two nostrils.

Complication A condition that occurs as the result of another disease or condition. It may also be an unwanted side-effect of treatment.

Composite lift Surgery to lift the skin and underlying soft tissues of the face, the brow and the upper eyelids.

Congenital Present from birth.

Conjunctiva The mucous membrane that covers the front of the eyeball and lines the eyelids.

Connective tissue Fibrous tissue that connects and supports organs within the body.

Consent form A form that patients must sign before surgery to confirm they understand what is involved in their operation and give their consent for it to take place. Signing the form also gives consent for the use of anaesthetic drugs and any other procedures which doctors feel to be necessary.

Contraindication Some condition or disease that makes it undesirable to give a treatment or medicine that would otherwise be given.

Cosmetic scar A scar that is relatively inconspicuous once it heals. Cosmetic scars are sometimes achieved by stitching the wound under the surface of the skin (subcuticular closure).

Cross-match Matching of donor and recipient blood to ensure that blood of the correct group is given on transfusion.

Cryotherapy The application of ice to reduce swelling, inflammation or bruising.

Cyst A fluid-filled swelling. Cysts can develop anywhere in the body as smooth, hard, sometimes painful lumps.

Day-case surgery Surgery for which a patient is in hospital for one day only, with no overnight stay.

Deep vein thrombosis (DVT) A blood clot in a deep vein, often in the lower leg or pelvis.

Dehiscence Complete breakdown of a wound causing it to gape open.

Dermabrasion Removal of the outer layer of the skin, often done with a small rotating instrument, to erase fine lines, small blemishes and scars. A similar process is involved in 'laser dermabrasion' although as the skin is not removed in this procedure, the term dermabrasion is not strictly correct.

Dermis The layer of skin below the epidermis.

Diagnosis The identification of a disease based on its symptoms and signs.

Diathermy A method of generating heat by means of a high-frequency electric current. It is used in surgery to destroy diseased tissue or to stop bleeding from damaged blood vessels.

Direct closure The drawing together of the edges of a wound with stitches.

Discharge letter A letter given to patients leaving hospital (or sent directly from the hospital) to deliver to their family doctor. It gives details of the treatment they have received and any follow-up required.

Dissect To separate structures by cutting or tearing the connective tissue that holds them together.

Diuretic Any substance that increases the volume of urine produced.

Divarication of the recti Separation or stretching of the vertical rectus muscles in the abdomen.

Donor site The part of the body from which tissues are taken to be grafted at another site to repair damage caused by disease, injury or surgery.

Drain/Drainage tube A tube that is inserted near a wound to drain excess blood and fluid into a bag or bottle.

Drip/Intravenous infusion A tube through which specially balanced saline or sugar solution is administered into a vein in the arm to replace fluid lost from the body after an operation or injury.

Dry eye syndrome Inflammation, soreness and dryness of the eye that may need to be treated by the insertion of artificial tears.

Ectropion Eversion of the lower eyelid resulting in functional disorder. It is a more serious version of scleral show.

Electrocardiogram (ECG) The activity of the heart recorded as a series of electrical wave patterns.

Electrocautery The application of the electrically heated tip of an instrument to the ends of blood vessels to stop them bleeding.

Embolus (plural: **emboli**) A piece of a blood clot (or air bubble) that has broken away and can pass through the blood vessels. If it lodges in a vital organ, such as the lung, it can have fatal consequences.

Endonasal rhinoplasty Surgery to change the shape or size of the nose that is performed through incisions made inside the nostrils; internal rhinoplasty.

Endoscope An instrument comprising a fibre-optic telescope, a bright light source, a channel through which fluid can be introduced or removed, and a channel through which other surgical instruments can be inserted.

Endoscopic surgery Surgery involving the insertion of an endoscope through small incisions, allowing the surgeon to view the operating site on a video or television monitor in the operating theatre.

Epidermis The outer cellular layer of the skin.

Epiphora Watering of the eyes due to excessive secretion from, or blockage of, the lacrimal ducts.

Erythema Redness due to increased blood flow.

Excision Removal by cutting.

External rhinoplasty See **Open rhinoplasty**.

Face lift An operation to tighten the skin, and possibly also the underlying soft tissues, of the face.

Familial Occurring in members of a family.

Fibrosis The development of excessive fibrous tissue.

Fixed Price Care The system used by some private hospitals whereby a fixed price is quoted for a particular type of operation and some of the hospitalisation costs associated with it.

Foreign body reaction The body's reaction to the presence of some substance which is not usually found within it. Large inflammatory cells accumulate around the foreign material in an attempt to seal it off and isolate it.

FRCS Fellow of the Royal College of Surgeons.

Gastrointestinal tract The stomach and intestines.

General anaesthetic A drug that induces loss of consciousness and abolishes the sensation of pain in all parts of the body.

Gland An organ that produces substances such as enzymes and hormones.

Goretex A substance more widely known for its use in the waterproofing of wet-weather gear, but that also has surgical uses, for example as an implant material in lip surgery.

Graft A piece of tissue removed from one site and placed at another to repair a defect resulting from an operation, accident or disease. The tissue can be taken from the same or another individual.

Haematoma A blood-filled swelling. A haematoma can form in a wound after an operation if blood continues to leak from a blood vessel. (If the blood spreads in the tissues, it appears as a bruise.)

Haemoglobin An iron-containing pigment in red blood cells that carries oxygen molecules around the body. As a good supply of oxygen is vital for wound healing, it is important that there is an adequate level of haemoglobin in the blood after surgery.

Haemophilia An inherited disease, transmitted by women but normally affecting only men, in which the mechanism of blood clotting is faulty, leading to uncontrolled bleeding when a blood vessel is severed.

Haemorrhage Bleeding.

Heparin A substance that occurs naturally in the body and helps prevent the blood clotting. It may be given by injection before and after surgery to people who are at particular risk of developing blood clots.

Hormone replacement therapy (HRT) Treatment with hormones that is given to women as their levels of oestrogen and progesterone fall before and after the menopause. It is now considered an important means of combatting the risk of brittle bones that can cause serious problems in elderly women.

Hyalin A material derived from collagen and deposited in the body around blood vessels and scars.

Hyperpigmentation An excess of pigment in the skin.

Hyperplasia Any condition in which there is an increase in the normal number of cells in a part of the body, causing enlargement.

Hypoplasia Defective development or underdevelopment of a tissue or body part.

Incision A cut or wound made by a sharp instrument, such as during an operation.

Incontinence Lack of voluntary control over the discharge of urine or faeces.

Induction agent A drug used in anaesthesia to bring on loss of consciousness.

Inflammation The response of a tissue to injury or infection that involves the rush of blood and white blood cells to the affected part, causing redness, swelling and pain.

Inhalational anaesthetic An anaesthetic given as a mixture of gases that is inhaled, usually to maintain anaesthesia.

Internal rhinoplasty See **Endonasal rhinoplasty**.

Intra-operative Occurring during an operation.

Intravenous anaesthetic A general anaesthetic drug that is injected via a cannula into a vein, usually in the back of the hand.

Keloid The overgrowth of fibrous tissue in a scar.

Langer's line A natural crease line in the skin. Incisions can sometimes be made along one of these lines so that the resulting scar is less obvious.

Laser A device that emits a visible or invisible beam of great intensity which can be precisely directed and controlled.

Laser skin resurfacing A form of dermabrasion using lasers that are controlled by computer; laser dermabrasion.

Lipectomy Excision of excess fatty tissue.

Liposculpture A procedure involving liposuction of superficial fat deposits plus the injection of fat to smooth the body's contours.

Liposuction The use of suction to remove excess fatty tissue, usually from deep under the skin.

Local anaesthetic An anaesthetic that numbs the area of the body around which it is injected.

Local injection An injection of a substance that remains confined to one area and is not distributed throughout the body.

Lymph A pale-coloured fluid that flows within the lymphatic vessels of the body and is eventually returned to the blood. It contains disease-fighting cells called lymphocytes.

Magnetic resonance imaging (MRI) The use of a large magnet to produce a magnetic field in individual cells of the body. An energy field is applied which affects the alignment of atoms within the cells and causes them to emit a signal which is detected by a computer and interpreted as an image of the body. This scanning procedure is very useful for visualising soft tissues that are not seen on routine X-rays.

Maintenance agent A drug used during an operation to maintain the state of general anaesthesia.

Mammaplasty Surgery to alter the shape and/or size of the breasts.

Mammography X-ray examination of the soft tissues of the breasts.

Mask face lift An operation involving lifting of all the facial structures, including the deep soft tissues and muscle.

Mastectomy Surgical removal of a breast, and usually also of the lymph nodes in the armpit.

Mastopexy Surgery to lift drooping breasts.

Medical history The record of someone's past health, including diseases, operations, allergies etc.

Menopause The time in a woman's life when her menstrual periods cease. It signals the end of her reproductive ability and may be associated with troublesome symptoms.

Mesotherapy A procedure more commonly used to treat arthritis in some countries but which is sometimes also used to treat cellulite. It involves a series of weekly injections of drugs into the fat beneath the skin.

Mini face lift A limited operation to tighten the skin of the face, leaving the deeper soft tissues untouched.

Mini tummy tuck An operation to remove fat and skin from the abdomen which, unlike a conventional tummy tuck, does not involve relocation of the umbilicus.

Monitoring device Equipment that is used to watch over the various activities of the body, such as the heart rate, pulse etc.

Nasal septum The central wall separating the two sides of the nose.

Nasolabial fold The fold of skin and soft tissue between the nose and upper lip.

National Health Service (NHS) The system of medical care, set up in Britain in 1948, under which medical treatment is mostly funded by taxation. NHS funding is not available for the majority of cosmetic operations.

Nausea A feeling of sickness.

Necrosis The death of tissue.

Nerve palsy Loss of function in some part of the body due to damage to its nerves.

Neuroma A swelling of nerve cells and nerve fibres.

Nil by mouth A term used to mean that no food or drink should be swallowed in the hours before an operation.

Nipple The projection from the areola of the breast on which the lactiferous ducts open.

Nodule A small swelling of cells.

Obesity An excessive amount of fat in the body. This term is non-specific and is being replaced by a figure calculated from height and weight measurements, known as the **body mass index**.

Oedema Swelling caused by an excessive amount of fluid in the spaces between the cells of tissues. It may occur as a result of inflammation, an allergic reaction, or obstruction of the lymphatic or blood vessels.

Oestrogen A hormone that stimulates sexual development in women at puberty and changes in the lining of the womb during the menstrual cycle.

Open rhinoplasty Surgery to the nose that involves an external incision being made across the vertical strut between the two nostrils; external rhinoplasty.

Orbital septum A thin sheet of connective tissue between the arch of bone above the eye and the muscles of the upper and lower eyelids.

Otoplasty Pinnaplasty.

Palpation Physical examination using the hands.

Patient-controlled analgesia (PCA) The administration of pain-killing drugs via a cannula inserted into a vein in the hand or arm, which is controlled by the patient. A preset dosage of the drug is delivered by a pump whenever the patient presses a button on the PCA machine.

Peri-areolar incision An incision made around the pigmented areola.

Pinna The external part of the ear.

Pinnaplasty Plastic surgery to the outer ear to correct deformity; otoplasty.

Plication A surgical process involving making tucks or pleats.

Poland's syndrome A condition affecting the hand and pectoralis muscle on one side of the body that is associated with failure of the breast on that side to grow normally.

Post-menopausal Following the menopause.

Post-operative Following an operation.

Pre-medication ('Pre-med.') A drug that is given before another drug, for example one given an hour or two prior to surgery to relax the patient before anaesthesia is started.

Pre-operative Before an operation.

Pre-operative assessment/Pre-clerking admission procedure A procedure used in some hospitals whereby patients attend an appointment a few days or weeks before an operation for any necessary pre-operative tests, such as blood tests and ECGs, the results of which are thus available by the time they are admitted for surgery.

Proptosis Bulging of the eyeball; a rare but serious complication following blepharoplasty.

Ptosis Drooping of an organ.

Pulmonary embolism A blood clot or air bubble blocking the blood vessels in the lung.

Pus A liquid produced as a result of inflammation. It contains both dead and living tissue fragments, cells and bacteria.

Pyrexia A fever.

Recovery room A ward near the operating theatre to which patients are taken after surgery so that they can be closely watched while they recover from a general anaesthetic.

Rectus muscle The vertical strap of muscle on either side of the midline in the abdomen.

Reduction mammaplasty Surgery to reduce the size of the breast(s).

Reduction rhinoplasty Surgery to reduce the size of the nose by reshaping its bone and cartilage through incisions made inside the nostrils.

Regional anaesthesia Anaesthesia of a specific area of the body.

Resect To cut out a portion of a tissue or organ.

Retin A A cream containing the vitamin-A derivative tretinoin. It was originally developed for the treatment of acne but was found to improve the appearance of fine wrinkles and the signs of sun damage in the skin. It encourages the production of new cells in the lower layer of the epidermis as well as the loss of old, dead cells from the skin's surface.

Retinova A variation of Retin A cream.

Retrobulbar haematoma A blood-filled swelling behind the eyeball.

Rhinitis Inflammation of the mucosal membrane of the nose that causes it to 'run'.

Rhinoplasty   Surgery to alter the size and/or shape of the nose.

Rhytidectomy   Literally, the excision of wrinkles, but it is also the name given to an operation to tighten the skin of the face, and possibly also the underlying soft tissues; a face lift.

Saline   A solution containing common salt. Saline solution has various medical uses, and is the filler in some types of breast implant.

Sclera   The outer, white, opaque coat of the eyeball that maintains its shape.

Scleral show   A condition in which an abnormal amount of the white of the eye (the **sclera**) is visible beneath the cornea due to drooping of the lower eyelid.

Sclerotherapy   Injection of a chemical into a vein that causes its walls to stick together, thus preventing the passage of blood through it.

Sedative   A substance that reduces the activity of a tissue, organ or entire organism, particularly the nervous system.

Sepsis   Infection caused by pus-producing bacteria.

Septicaemia   Severe infection caused by large numbers of bacteria in the blood that multiply and spread; blood poisoning.

Septoplasty   Surgery to adjust the bone between the two nostrils and thus improve breathing through the nose.

Seroma   A collection of clear fluid, such as lymph, which may develop following an operation. If persistent, the fluid can be drawn off with a needle.

Sickle cell anaemia   A severe, sometimes fatal, form of anaemia resulting from the presence in red blood cells of an abnormal type of haemoglobin that causes them to become crescent (or sickle) shaped. It is a familial condition, most common in negroid races.

Side-effect   An effect other than that desired, resulting from the use of a drug or other form of treatment.

Sign   Something a doctor looks for as an indication of disease, such as redness or swelling.

Silicone A compound made from the organic substance silicon. It can be in the form of an oil, grease or solid and has numerous uses, including many medical ones.

SMAS face lift An operation to lift the skin of the face together with the underlying soft tissues and muscle of the superficial musculo-aponeurotic system (SMAS).

Spider veins A term often (mis)used to cover a wide variety of superficial blood vessel abnormalities.

Step-down ward A ward to which day-case patients are taken in some hospitals to recover before going home after surgery.

Steroid One of a group of naturally occurring substances in the body that includes some hormones.

Subareolar incision An incision made at the junction of the pigmented area and the rest of the skin of the breast.

Subcutaneous Under the skin.

Subcuticular Under the upper layer of the skin.

Submammary incision An incision made in the crease underneath the breast; inframammary incision.

Supraorbital rim The rim of bone above the eye, just below the eyebrow.

Suture A surgical stitch or row of stitches.

Symptom Something experienced by a patient that indicates a disturbance of normal body function, for example pain or nausea.

Testosterone A hormone secreted by the testes that promotes the growth and function of the secondary male characteristics.

Thalassaemia A group of disorders caused by an inherited defect in the structure of haemoglobin involving a chronic, progressive form of anaemia. It is most common in races from the Mediterranean area, Middle East and Far East.

Thrombo-embolic deterrent stockings (TEDS) See **Anti-embolism stockings**.

Thrombophlebitis Inflammation of a vein following the formation of a blood clot within it.

Thromboplastin   A substance that is released into the bloodstream when blood is shed and that plays a role in the formation of a blood clot.

Thrombosis   The coagulation of blood within a vein or artery that produces a blood clot.

Thrombus   A blood clot that remains within the blood vessel in which it forms.

Toxicity   The quality of being poisonous.

Tracheal tube   A tube that is inserted into the windpipe (the **trachea**) to keep the airways to the lungs open during anaesthesia; an endotracheal tube.

Tragus   The projection of cartilage in front of the external opening of the ear.

Trauma   Injury.

Triglyceride   A substance present in most animal and vegetable fats. It is used as a filler in some types of breast implant, and has the advantage of being absorbed and digested by the body should leakage occur.

Tumescent liposuction   The treatment of cellulite using liposuction following the injection of a mixture of saline, local anaesthetic, adrenaline and a drug called hyalase; wet liposuction.

Tummy tuck   Surgery to remove fat and excess skin from the lower abdomen; abdominoplasty.

Ultrasound/Ultrasonography   Examination of the soft tissues of the body that involves the passage of high-frequency sound waves. The waves are reflected back from any solid object, much like an echo, and, once processed by a computer, can be used to build up a picture of an area of tissue.

Umbilicus   The navel.

Urinalysis   The analysis of urine to detect the presence of certain chemicals and/or of bacteria.

Urinary catheter   A narrow tube inserted through the urethra into the bladder to drain urine from it. It may be used for a short period after surgery until urine can be passed spontaneously again.

Urinary retention   Retention of urine in the bladder caused by obstruction to its flow or weakness of the muscles of the bladder wall.

Warfarin   An anticoagulant that may be used in the treatment of thrombosis to thin the blood and help dissolve a blood clot.

Wet liposuction   Tumescent liposuction.

X-ray   A type of electromagnetic radiation of short wavelength that is able to pass through opaque bodies. It can be used in diagnosis, by allowing the visualisation of internal structures and organs of the body, or in higher doses as therapy to destroy malignant cells.

Useful addresses

There are organisations in most countries throughout the world that provide advice, information and, in som cases, practical support, both for those considering cosmetic surgery and for those having to come to terms with disfigurement of some sort. A few examples are listed here; details of others may be found in local telephone directories or can be obtained from hospitals or health departments.

British Association of Aesthetic Plastic Surgeons
Royal College of Surgeons
35 Lincoln's Inn Fields
London WC2A 3PN
Telephone: 0171 405 2234
Information sheets are available with details of different cosmetic procedures. The association can also provide a list of accredited cosmetic plastic surgeons on receipt of a stamped, addressed envelope.

British Association of Plastic Surgeons
Royal College of Surgeons
35 Lincoln's Inn Fields
London WC2A 3PN
Telephone: 0171 831 5161/5162
Information is available about plastic surgery for burns and reconstruction.

General Medical Council
44 Hallam Street
London W1N 6AE
Telephone: 0171 580 7642

Enquiries can be made about whether a particular surgeon is on the specialist register of plastic surgeons, and thus recognised by the GMC as being suitably accredited.

Outlook
Disfigurement Support Unit
Ward 22
Frenchay Hospital
Bristol BS16 1LE
Telephone: 0117 9753889
Outlook offers support and assistance to anyone needing help to come to terms with a disfigurement or unusual physical characteristic. This is an NHS service open to adults and children, who must be referred by their family doctor, consultant or school doctor. Assessment is made by a clinical psychologist and a whole range of group and individual sessions is run to help people cope with difficulties arising from disfigurement such as cleft lip, burn scars, birthmarks, skin problems etc.

Changing Faces
Telephone: 0171 251 4232
This is a London-based charity that offers an information service to deal with questions about all types of facial disfigurement.

Disfigurement Guidance Centre
P.O. Box 7
Cupar
Fife KY15 4PF
Telephone: 01227 870281
The centre publishes a guide to laser treatment, both NHS and private, in its *Skin Laser Directory*. It also produces a *National Disfigurement Register* providing information about treatment, self-help groups and a range of camouflaging and corrective cosmetics.

British Association of Skin Camouflage
C/O Mrs J. Goulding
25 Blackhorse Drive
Silkstone Common
Barnsley
South Yorkshire S75 4SD
Telephone: 01226 790744
Information about the services offered is available on receipt of a stamped, addressed envelope. Advice about appropriate cover-up creams and make-ups can be given by local members for a small fee.

AUSTRALIA

Royal Australasian College of Surgeons
Division of Plastic and Reconstructive Surgery
College of Surgeons Gardens
Spring Street
Melbourne
Victoria 3000
Australia
Telephone: 03 92491200

NEW ZEALAND

Royal Australasian College of Surgeons
P.O. Box 7451
Wellington South
Wellington
New Zealand
Telephone: 04 3858247

CANADA

Canadian Society of Plastic Surgeons
Suite 520
30 Boulevard St Joseph East
Montreal
Quebec H2T 1G9
Canada
Telephone: 514 843 5415

USA

American Association of Plastic Surgeons
10666 N. Torrey Pines Road
La Jolla
California 92037
USA
Telephone: 619 554 9940

American Society for Aesthetic Plastic Surgery
3922 Atlantic Avenue
Long Beach
California 90807
USA
Telephone: 310 595 4275

American Society of Plastic and Reconstructive Surgeons
444 E. Algonquin Road
Arlington Heights
Illinois 60005
USA
Telephone: 708 228 9900

APPENDIX VI

How to complain

If you are unhappy about any aspect of your treatment or care, the best approach in the first instance is to make a polite and reasoned enquiry to the person concerned, who may be able to deal with your complaint immediately. However angry or irritated you may feel, a complaint made aggressively is unlikely to achieve much. If you are not happy with the response you receive, you can then consider pursuing your complaint through the various paths that exist to deal with such problems.

Before you set the complaints machinery in motion, however, it is worth thinking carefully about what is involved. Once a formal complaint has been made against a doctor and the complaints procedure has begun, there is little chance of stopping it. The vast majority of doctors are dedicated, conscientious and hard working, and really do have their patients' best interests at heart. A complaint against a doctor is usually a devastating blow, which can cause considerable stress. Of course, if something has gone wrong during your treatment, you may also have suffered stress and unhappiness, but before you make an official complaint, do consider whether your doctor's actions have really warranted what many would see as a 'kick in the teeth'.

Details of all the appropriate councils and complaints procedures and how they work can be obtained from your hospital or local health authority. If you have any problems with the offices mentioned below, information about what to do and who to go to for help is available from Citizens' Advice Bureaus and Community Health Councils.

Individual consultants are responsible for all aspects of the care of their patients when receiving treatment in a private hospital, and private patients should therefore approach their consultants in the first instance if they have a complaint to make. However, like doctors employed by the NHS, private consultants are also ultimately answerable to their own professional bodies.

HOSPITAL STAFF

If your complaint concerns something that has happened during your stay in hospital and for some reason you are unable to approach the person directly concerned, you can talk to the ward sister or charge nurse, the hospital doctor on your ward, or the senior manager for the department or ward. If they cannot deal with your complaint directly, they will be able to refer you to the appropriate person.

THE GENERAL MANAGER

If you are intimidated by the thought of speaking to one of the people mentioned above, you can write to the hospital's General Manager, sometimes called the Director of Operations or Chief Executive. The General Manager has responsibility for the way the hospital is run. If you would prefer to do so, you can make an appointment to speak to him or her, rather than writing a letter.

The Patients' Charter states that anyone making a complaint about an NHS service must receive a 'full and prompt written reply from the Chief Executive or General Manager'. You should therefore receive an immediate response to your letter, and your complaint should be fully investigated by a senior manager. Depending on how serious your complaint is, you should then receive either a full report of the investigation into it or regular letters telling you what is happening until such a report can be made. Do make sure you keep copies of all letters you write and receive.

DISTRICT HEALTH AUTHORITY

If the treatment you require is not available in your area, or the waiting list is very long, your local District Health Authority may be able to arrange for you to have treatment elsewhere where waiting lists are shorter, if this is what you want. The District Health Authority is able to deal with complaints concerning the provision of services, rather than with those resulting from something going wrong with your treatment.

COMMUNITY HEALTH COUNCIL

Independent advice and assistance can be obtained from your local Community Health Council. Someone from the Community Health Council will be able to explain the complaints procedures to you, help you to write letters to the hospital, and also come with you to any meetings arranged between hospital representatives and yourself.

REGIONAL MEDICAL OFFICER

If your complaint concerns the standard of *clinical* treatment you received in hospital, and the paths you have already taken have not led to a satisfactory conclusion, you can take it to the Regional Medical Officer for your area.

FAMILY HEATLH SERVICES AUTHORITY

Family doctors are now encouraged to have their own 'in-house' complaints services, but a complaint about your family doctor that you have been unable to sort out by this means can be reported to the Family Health Services Authority. Such complaints should be made within 13 weeks of the incident occurring. Again, your local Community Health Council will be able to give you advice and help you make your complaint and write letters etc.

HEALTH SERVICE COMMISSIONER

If all else has failed, you can take your complaint to the Health Service Commissioner, who is responsible to Parliament and independent of both the NHS and the government.

The Health Service Commissioner can deal with complaints made by individuals about the failure of an NHS authority to provide the service it should – a failure that has caused actual hardship or injustice – but is not able to investigate complaints about clinical treatment. You must have taken your complaint up with your local health authority first, but if you have not received a satisfactory response within a reasonable time, write to the Health Service Commissioner enclosing copies of *all* the relevant letters and documents as well as giving details of the incident itself.

You must contact the Health Service Commissioner within *one year* of the incident occurring, unless there is some valid reason why you have been unable to do so.

There is a separate Health Service Commissioner for each country within the United Kingdom.

Health Service Commissioner for England
Church House
Great Smith Street
London SW1P 3BW
Telephone: 0171 276 2035

Health Service Commissioner for Scotland
Second Floor, 11 Melville Crescent
Edinburgh EH3 7LU
Telephone: 0131 225 7465

Health Service Commissioner for Wales
4th Floor Pearl Assurance House
Greyfriars Road
Cardiff CF1 3AG
Telephone: 01222 394621

Office of the Northern Ireland Commissioner for Complaints
33 Wellington Place
Belfast BT1 6HN
Telephone: 01232 233821

TAKING LEGAL ACTION

The legal path is likely to be an expensive one, and should be a last resort rather than a starting point.

In theory, everyone has a right to take legal action. However, unless you have very little money and are entitled to Legal Aid, or a great deal of money, you are unlikely to be able to afford this costly process. The outcome of legal action can never be assured, and the possible cost if you lose your case should be borne in mind.

If you do think you have grounds for compensation for injury caused to you as a result of negligence, advice can be sought from:

The Association for the Victims of Medical Accidents (AVMA)
1 London Road
Forest Hill
London SE23 3TP
Telephone: 0181 291 2793.

Someone from the AVMA will be able to give you free and confidential legal advice about whether or not you have a case worth pursuing and will be able to recommend solicitors with training in medical law who may be prepared to represent you.

Index

abdominoplasty (tummy tuck) 86–91
  and liposuction 82
abnormality
  congenital 3, 65
  medical 5
abscess 98
admission to hospital 28–9
ageing, signs of 37
  on breasts 69, 81
  on brow 47
  on facial skin 43
  on lips 62
  on skin around eyes 50
  reversing 4, 5
alar cartilage 58
allergic reactions
  to anaesthetics 6, 17–18
  to collagen injections 63
anaemia
  after liposuction 86
  blood test for 19
anaesthesia
  general 106–109
    administration of 33–4
    and false teeth 31–2
    driving and 31
    risks of 108–109
    side–effects of 108
  local 105–106, 107
    administration of 33
  nerve block 106
anaesthetic room 33–4
anaesthetist 28, 105
  ward visit by 30–31
analgesia, patient
    controlled 109–110

analgesics 28, *see also* painkillers
anticoagulants 30, 97, 101
anti-embolism stockings 29–30, 87, 101–102
anti-emetics 107
aspirin, risks of with
    mammaplasty 71, 76
asymmetry
  after augmentation
    mammaplasty 75
  after brow lift 49
  after pinnaplasty 68
  after reduction mammaplasty 80
  after rhytidectomy 46
augmentation mammaplasty 70–75

'bat ears' 65
bipolar diathermy 23
bleeding
  controlling during surgery 23
  post-operative 97
    after blepharoplasty 56
    after liposuction 86
    after pinnaplasty 67
    after rhinoplasty 61
blepharoplasty 50–56
  and laser dermabrasion 40
blindness, risk of after eyelid
    surgery 53–4
blood clot, *see* thrombus
blood pressure, and anaesthesia 107
blood tests 19–20
blood transfusion 20
  after liposuction 86
  after reduction mammaplasty 78
Board Certified Plastic Surgeon 8

breast implants 69–70
  and mastopexy 81
  insertion of 71
  movement of 74
    and asymmetry 75
  protrusion of 75
  removal of 74, 75
  rupture of 74–5
  saline-filled 73
  silicone 70
  wrinkling of 74
breast lift, *see* mastopexy
breastfeeding
  after augmentation mammaplasty 73
  after reduction mammaplasty 79
breasts
  effects of age on 69, 81
  growth of 69, 70, 76
breast surgery
  augmentation mammaplasty 69, 70–75
  mastopexy 69, 81
  reduction mammaplasty 69, 76–80
British Association of Aesthetic Plastic Surgeons (BAAPS) 8
British Association of Plastic Surgeons (BAPS) 8
brow lift 47–9
bruising 96
  after abdominoplasty 89
  after brow lift 49
  after liposuction 85
  after lip surgery 64
  after pinnaplasty 67
  after rhinoplasty 60
  after rhytidectomy 45
  and haematoma 97

cannula
  for administration of anaesthetic 33–4
  for liposuction 83–5
capsular contracture 74
  and breast asymmetry 75
cartilage
  alar 58
  folding of in pinna 65, 66, 67

cellulite, treatment of 91
cellulitis 90
cellulolipolysis 91
chemical peel 38–9
chest infection 101
children
  and cosmetic surgery 4, 16
  and pinnaplasty 65
collagen injections 62–3
columella 59
complications, post-operative
  general 93–102
  of abdominoplasty 90–91
  of augmentation mammaplasty 73–5
  of blepharoplasty 53–6
  of brow lift 49
  of collagen injections 63
  of Goretex insertion 63
  of liposuction 85–6
  of mastopexy 81
  of pinnaplasty 67–8
  of reduction mammaplasty 79
  of rhinoplasty 61
  of rhytidectomy 46–7
composite face lift 44
consent forms 30
consultant, *see* surgeon
contraceptive pill 18
  and liposuction 83
  and mammaplasty 71
cosmetic clinics 10–11

day-case surgery 21, 108
deep vein thrombosis 101–102, *see also* thrombosis
depression, post-operative 14
  after rhytidectomy 45
dermabrasion 39, *see also* laser dermabrasion
diathermy 23
divarication of the recti 89
doctor
  family, referral by 6
  hospital, ward visit by 30
doctors, hospital 26–8
double vision, after blepharoplasty 53

INDEX

driving
  after augmentation mammaplasty 73
  after blepharoplasty 53
  after general anaesthesia 31
drooping, *see* ptosis
drugs 31
  and hospital admission 23
  non-prescription 18
dry eye syndrome 55

ears
  prominent 65
  surgery, *see* pinnaplasty
ectropion 56
electrocardiogram 19
  and anaesthesia 106–107
embolus 102
emergency facilities 10
endonasal (internal) rhinoplasty 58
  complications of 61
  post-operative care 60–61
endoscope 35
endoscopic surgery 35
  augmentation mammaplasty 73
  brow lift 47, 49
  face lift 44
epiphora 54
ERBIUM:YAG lasers 40
external rhinoplasty, *see* open rhinoplasty
eyeball, bulging of 56
eyelid surgery, *see* blepharoplasty

face, effects of age on 37
face lift, *see* rhytidectomy
fat removal 82–91
Fellow of the Royal College of Surgeons (FRCS) 8
Fixed Price Care 113
fluid, collection of 99

general anaesthesia, *see* anaesthesia
General Medical Council (GMC) 7
Goretex, use of in lips 63
grafts
  for nipple reconstruction 80
  for skin necrosis 99
  to augment lips 64

haematoma 97–8
  after abdominoplasty 90
  after blepharoplasty 53
  after liposuction 85
  after mammaplasty 79
  after pinnaplasty 67
  after rhytidectomy 46
  retrobulbar 56
hair, loss of
  after brow lift 49
  after rhytidectomy 46
health insurance, private 111–112
heparin, use of
  pre-operatively 30
  post-operatively 101, 102
  after abdominoplasty 87
hormone replacement therapy (HRT) 18
hyalin injections 62–3
hyperplasia 76
hypoplasia 70

implants, *see* breast implants
incisions
  for abdominoplasty 87–8
  for augmentation mammaplasty 71–3
  for blepharoplasty 51, 52
  for brow lift 48, 49
  for liposuction 83
  for mastopexy 81
  for pinnaplasty 66, 67
  for reduction mammaplasty 76, 77, 78
  for rhinoplasty 58, 59
  for rhytidectomy 43
induction agents 107
infection
  after abdominoplasty 90
  after augmentation mammaplasty 75
  after Goretex insertion 63
  after lip surgery 64
  after pinnaplasty 67
  and pain 97
  in chest 101
  in wound 98
inhalational anaesthetic 106
insurance, *see* health insurance

internal rhinoplasty, *see* endonasal rhinoplasty
intravenous anaesthetic 106

keloid scars 99–100
   after pinnaplasty 67

laser dermabrasion 40–41
laser skin resurfacing, *see* laser dermabrasion
lipectomy 82, *see also* abdominoplasty
liposuction 82–6
   and abdominoplasty 87
lip surgery 62, 64
local anaesthesia, *see* anaesthesia
lower eyelid surgery 52, *see also* blepharoplasty

maintenance agents 107
mammaplasty, *see* breast surgery
mask face lift 44
mastopexy 69, 81
mesotherapy 91
mini face lift 42
   and laser dermabrasion 40
mini tummy tuck 89
muscle relaxants 107
   post-operative effects of 108

named nurse 28
National Health Service (NHS) 21
   availability of treatment 3, 5
   cancellation of operations 32–3
   emergency facilities at hospitals 10
   treatment for pinnaplasty 65
neck lift 41–7
necrotising fasciitis 90, 98
nerve damage 100–101
   after rhytidectomy 46
nerve palsy 101
neuroma 100
'nil by mouth' 32
nipple
   change in sensation of
      after augmentation mammaplasty 75
      after reduction mammaplasty 80
   loss of after reduction mammaplasty 80
   reconstruction of after reduction mammaplasty 80
   repositioning of
      in mastopexy 81
      in reduction mammaplasty 78
nose
   bleeding after rhytidectomy 61
   reshaping of 57
   surgery, *see* rhinoplasty
numbness, *see* sensation, loss of
nursing staff 24–6

obesity, and risks of surgery 95
open rhinoplasty 59
   complications of 61
   post-operative care 60–61
operating department assistant 34, 106
operating theatre 34
   nurses in 24
operations, *see also* individual operations
   cancellation of 32–3
   complications of 95–102
   paying for 112–13
otoplasty, *see* pinnaplasty
oxygen, and wound healing 19

pain, post-operative 96–7, 105
painkillers 107
pinnaplasty (otoplasty) 65–8
Poland's syndrome 69
post-operative care
   after abdominoplasty 89
   after augmentation mammaplasty 73
   after blepharoplasty 53
   after brow lift 49
   after liposuction 85
   after reduction mammaplasty 78–9
   after rhinoplasty 60–61
   after rhytidectomy 44–5
pre-medication 31
pre-operative appointments 17–18
   for abdominoplasty 87

INDEX

for augmentation
  mammaplasty 71–2
for blepharoplasty 50–51
for brow lift 47
for liposuction 83
for pinnaplasty 65
for reduction mammaplasty 76–7
for rhinoplasty 57–8
for rhytidectomy 41–2
pre-operative tests 19–20, 29
  for blepharoplasty 51
private hospitals 10
proptosis 56
psychologist, referral to 17
ptosis
  of breasts 81
  of facial soft tissues 43–4
  of upper eyelid 54
pulmonary embolism 102
pyrexia 96

recovery room 107
  nurses in 24
reduction mammaplasty 76–80
reduction rhinoplasty 57–61
Retin A 37–8
retinoeic acid creams 37–8
Retinova 37–8
retrobulbar haematoma 56
rhinitis 61
rhinoplasty 57–61
rhytidectomy 41–7
  and liposuction 82

scars 99–100
  after abdominoplasty 87, 89–90
  after augmentation
    mammaplasty 71–2, 73, 74
  after blepharoplasty 53
    and scleral show 55
  after Goretex insertion 63
  after laser dermabrasion 41
  after liposuction 85, 86
  after lip surgery 64
  after mastopexy 81
  after pinnaplasty 67
  after reduction mammaplasty 76, 79, 80
  after rhinoplasty 57, 59

after rhytidectomy 46
  care of 100
scleral show 55
secondary rhinoplasty 61
sensation, loss of 100–101
  after abdominoplasty 91
  after augmentation
    mammaplasty 75
  after brow lift 49
  after liposuction 85
  after reduction mammaplasty 80
  after rhinoplasty 61
  after rhytidectomy 45, 46
septoplasty 57
seroma 99
  after abdominoplasty 90
  after liposuction 85
sexual intercourse, after reduction
    mammaplasty 80
silicone, in breast implants 70
skin loss/necrosis 99
  after abdominoplasty 90
  after reduction mammaplasty 80
  after rhytidectomy 46
SMAS face lift 43–4
smoking
  and chest infection 101
  and risks of surgery 96
sore throat, after general
    anaesthetic 108
spider veins
  after rhinoplasty 61
  after rhytidectomy 46
step-down ward 108
superficial liposculpture 91
surgeon
  choice of 7–8
  paying fees of 112
  ward visit by 30
surgeons 26–8
  at cosmetic clinics 10
  register of 7
  training and qualifications of 8, 9
surgery
  contraindications to 12–13, 16
  indications for 15
  restrictions on 11–12
swelling
  after abdominoplasty 89, 90

swelling, *continued*
  after augmentation mammaplasty 75
  after blepharoplasty 54, 55
  after liposuction 85
  after lip surgery 64
  after reduction mammaplasty 78–9
  after rhinoplasty 61
  after rhytidectomy 45

temperature, raised 96
  and haematoma 97–8
  and wound infection 98
tests, *see* pre-operative tests
thrombo-embolic deterrent stockings (TEDS), *see* anti-embolism stockings
thrombo-embolism and HRT 18
thrombophlebitis, after breast surgery 75
thrombosis 18, 101
  reducing the risks of 29–30
thrombus 18, 101–102
tumescent liposuction 83

tummy tuck, *see* abdominoplasty
typecasting 5–6

umbilicus, in abdominoplasty 87, 88, 89
upper eyelid surgery 51, *see also* blepharoplasty
urinalysis 20, 29
urinary catheter, use of after abdominoplasty 89

warfarin, for deep vein thrombosis 101
watering of the eyes, *see* epiphora
wound dehiscence 99
wound infection 98, *see also* infection
wounds, healing of 100
wrinkles, removal of on face
  with dermabrasion 39
  with laser dermabrasion 40
  with retinoeic acid creams 37
  with rhytidectomy 41

X-rays 19, 27